# AUTOPHAGY

*Learn How to Activate the Self-cleansing Process of Your Body and Improve Your Health with Intermittent Fasting and Ketosis*

**© Written By David Colombo**

# TABLE OF CONTENTS

# INTRODUCTION

Autophagy is the natural process by which our body removes out cellular junk to let new cell growth. It makes total sense that our body needs an internal clean up to detox and repair it self. Autophagy destroys parts of the cell, proteins and cell membranes which are not functioning properly. One good example of autophagy is losing appetite when we feel very sick. Most of us will just lie down for hours or days, without eating anything until we have substantially recuperated. In fact, Autophagy has been discovered to help cure and prevent a number of disease conditions. Even experts found a number of interesting clinical trials and studies of what autophagy and intermittent fasting can do to promote wellness and good health.

Autophagy is a key process that keeps your body's cells in proper balance, or what we call homeostasis. A popular saying about sustainability for the environment is "Reduce, reuse, recycle." In a lot of ways, autophagy is the natural process that does all three of these things for your body. The term "autophagy" comes from the Latin word that means "self-eating." This is because the process of autophagy breaks down parts of your cells in order to recycle them in the creation of new cells.

Cytoplasm consists of fluid inside of a cell (excluding the nucleus). During autophagy, cytoplasm and organelles (small structures with specific functions) are removed and recycled. This process keeps your body in balance by self-removing cells that are no longer functioning optimally or appropriately.

While autophagy helps to keep your body in balance, there are also disorders that disrupt normal processes of autophagy, which leads to chronic illness. Neurodegenerative disorders like Parkinson's disease have genetic links to being related to dysfunction in autophagy.

Autophagy has important effects that occur both within the cell and outside of the cell. Within the cell, autophagy helps to decrease oxidative stress, increase genomic stability (which aids in the prevention of cancer), increase bioenergetic metabolism, and increase the elimination of waste.

Outside of the cell, autophagy helps to decrease inflammatory response, increase neuroendocrine homeostasis, increase surveillance of cancer by the immune system, and increase elimination of aging cells.

# CHATER ONE
## UNDERSTANDING AUTOPHAGY

### The Origins of Autophagy

In the 1950s, Belgian scientist Christian de Duve was studying insulin when he accidentally discovered a process he called autophagy, from the Greek words for "self" (auto) and "eating" (phagy). It is the mechanism by which cells cannibalize some of their own parts in a continual cleanup process.

In the 1970s and '80s, researchers began looking at the process of autophagy. It had not been studied extensively at the time, and nobody really knew its role or why it was important. The big breakthrough came in 1983, when researcher Yoshinori Ohsumi, while conducting experiments in yeast, discovered the genes that regulate autophagy. He found that without those genes, autophagy doesn't work—and the cells can't repair themselves. He won the Nobel Prize in 2016, as his work was considered fundamentally important to understanding how autophagy functions in cells.

The most fascinating part of the discovery of autophagy is that the process is given a boost if there is cellular stress. If cells lack nutrients, are deprived of energy, or are damaged in some way, a "stress response" mechanism is activated, which initiates autophagy. As a result, cell function actually improves when we're under stress. In the absence of added stress, autophagy remains functioning at a moderate level, maintaining cell function. This is known as its maintenance mode.

The thinking goes that when you activate autophagy, you reduce the chance of developing age-related problems and thus extend your life span.

## Apoptosis

Let's talk death. What exactly is death? Death, for any organism, isn't one event. It's a series of small events that eventually piles up. And this death, like any death, is essential for life. For new life. Too far out? Allow me to explain. All organisms are large, complicated cellular structres. And cells within any organism (like our bodies) get damaged and die all the time. Old, damaged cells need to die, need to be wiped out, for new healthy cells to grow. It's a process that's continuously going on inside each one of us. Both at the cellular and the sub-cellular level.

## The What and How of Autophagy

Autophagy is a cellular pathway involved in protein and organelle degradation, which is likely to represent an innate adaptation to starvation. In times of nutrient deficiency, the cell can self-digest and recycle some nonessential components through nonselective autophagy, thus sustaining minimal growth requirements until a food source becomes available. "Auto" means self and "phagy" means eat. So the literal meaning of autophagy is "self-eating." Autophagy is when a cell consumes the parts of itself that are damaged or malfunctioning. Lysosomes, members of the innate immune system that also degrade pathogens—degrade the damaged cellular material, making it available for energy and other metabolites. Autophagy is the body's way of cleaning out damaged cells, in order to regenerate newer, healthier cells.

"When your cells get old or die, other cells clean them up and recycle the materials to build new, younger and healthier cells," Way explains, noting that without autophagy, "Our body would become a landfill, crammed with broken pieces or worse it would just shut down because nothing would be replaced." This cleanup can include anything from older and possibly cancerous cells to old skin cells, paving the way for the production of new ones.

Autophagy can also target excess fat. Specifically, according to information published in Scientific Report, autophagy may facilitate the conversion of the harmful white fat many of us are constantly trying to reduce into more metabolically sound brown fat, which contains countless energy-producing mitochondria and has been linked to lowering the risk of metabolic disease and diabetes. Autophagy can even help renew the neurons in the brain, improving energy and mood.

## PROCESS

Autophagy is typically triggered by a cell's starvation of nutrients. It is believed that insulin suppresses autophagy while glucagon can activate the process.

After eating, your body releases insulin, while fasting causes a release of glucagon as your body's blood sugar starts to decrease. Glucagon signals your body to use glycogen in your liver to increase your blood sugar. Once autophagy is activated, the process occurs in four steps.

- **Sequestration.** During this step, two membranes (called phagophore) elongate around and eventually enclose cytoplasm and organelles that are later to be degraded. This double-membrane becomes an organelle known as an autophagosome. Typically, the contents engulfed by the autophagosome are selected because they are within range. However, autophagosomes can be selective as the membrane can initiate autophagy when there is interaction with certain proteins in the cell.

- **Transport to a lysosome.** The autophagosomes cannot directly connect to a lysosome, so it first fuses with an intermediate structure called an endosome. The autophagosome that is fused with an endosome is now referred to as an amphisome, which can readily fuse with a lysosome.

- **Degradation.** This can begin after fusion with a lysosome occurs. Upon fusing with the amphisome, the lysosome releases enzymes (known as hydrolases) that degrade the materials that were in the original autophagosome. This structure that is full of degraded cellular material is now known as either an autolysosome or an autophagolysosome.

- **Utilization of degradation products.** This can occur after all cellular materials are degraded down to amino acids. After being exported out of the autolysosome into the cellular fluid, the amino acids can then be reused.

The fourth and final stage is ultimately related to the starvation of cellular nutrients. The utilization of degradation products is ultimately needed for providing amino acids for gluconeogenesis (a process in which the body synthesizes glucose from non-carbohydrate sources). The amino acids serve as an energy source for the tricarboxylic (TCA) cycle, and these amino acids can be recycled into synthesizing new proteins.

## Types of Autophagy

There are three types of autophagy. Although similar, they each have distinct features to differentiate each type.

- Macroautophagy

- Microautophagy

- Chaperone-mediated autophagy.

## Macroautophagy

The mechanism of macroautophagy is conserved among eukaryotes and is characterized by the encapsulation of cellular cargo into double-membrane vesicles called autophagosomes. In yeast, the formation of autophagosomes around the targeted cargo is mediated by autophagy-related (Atg) proteins that are recruited hierarchically to the phagophore assembly site or the preautophagosomal structure (PAS). At the PAS, initiator protein complexes facilitate the de novo synthesis of a double membrane structure called a phagophore or an isolation membrane, the lipid components for which are derived from the golgi-endosome system. In mammals, where a distinct PAS-like structure has not been identified, multiple cellular organelles, including the plasma membrane are known to serve as origins for the assembly of a phagophore. Upon the recruitment of other Atg proteins, the isolation membrane gets extended into a phagophore, which eventually fuses at its free ends to form an autophagosome, which now surrounds and sequesters the cargo. Once formed, autophagosomes undergo a maturation process as they are transported along the endocytic pathway, before fusing with the lysosomes to form autophagolysosomes. The cellular cargo delivered by the autophagosomes are then degraded by the hydrolytic enzymes of the lysosomes and the products of degradation are released back into the cytoplasm for cell use.

**Microautophagy**

Microautophagy is important in the maintenance of organellar size, membrane homeostats and cell survival under nitrogen restriction. In this process, lysosomes do not fuse with autophagic vesicles but directly engulf cytosoplasmic cargos (selectively, using chaperones or "in bulk") via invaginations of the lysosomal membrane. Next, there is vesicle scission into the lysosomal lumen, and degradation of the content occurs inside the lysosomes. In yeast, microautophagy is constitutive, but it can also be induced by starvation or treatment with rapamycin (an mTOR inhibitor drug). Similar to macroautophagy, microautophagy functions also as a "housekeeping" mechanism for the degradation of cytosolic materials. Microautophagy can occur simultaneously with macroautophagy to regulate lysosomal membrane size. As macroautophagy can result in a large flow of membranes to lysosomes, microautophagy can regulate this flow and reduce lysosomal size by consuming lysosomal membranes. Additionally, microautophagy was shown to play an important role in early mammalian development. Indeed, microautophagy was used to deliver endosomes to lysosomes in the visceral endoderm of mouse embryos. This process was found to be important for the proper delivery of maternal nutrients as well as signaling molecules to the embryo.

## Chaperone-mediated autophagy (CMA)

Chaperone-mediated autophagy (CMA) is a selective form of autophagy with distinctive mechanisms for cargo recognition and internalization into the lysosomal lumen. Only proteins amenable to unfolding can be internalized in lysosomes by CMA through a mechanism with resemblance to protein transport systems into other organelles such as mitochondria or ER.

CMA starts with binding of hsc70 to a consensus pentapeptide motif in the substrate protein. Hsc70 targets these proteins to the lysosomal membrane, and after binding to the cytosolic tail of LAMP2A (lysosome-associated membrane protein type 2A), the substrate proteins are unfolded and translocated oneby-one into the lysosomal lumen.

Transport through the membrane requires multimerization of LAMP2A into the CMA translocation complex and a form of hsc70 resident in the lysosomal lumen required to

complete substrate translocation. The substrates are then rapidly degraded in the lysosomal lumen. While effectors of other forms of autophagy are conserved from yeast to mammals,

LAMP2A, the essential CMA component, appears late in evolution. LAMP2A is a spliced variant of the lamp2 gene, absent in yeast, fungi and worms. A gene with homology to the mammalian lamp2 gene has been identified in Drosophila but with a c-terminus homologous to LAMP-2C but there is no evidence of splicing. In Zebrafish the two lamp2 variants described show higher homology to the mammalian LAMP2B and C variants. The LAMP2A exon has so far been described only in birds and mammals CMA, as the other components of the cellular proteostasis networks, does not function in isolation. Blockage of

15

CMA in vitro and in vivo is compensated for by upregulation of macroautophagy and of the proteasome system in most cell types. Conversely, cells respond to inhibition of macroautophagy or the proteasome by constitutively activating CMA. In most cases, compensation assures maintenance of cellular quality control and the energetic balance under basal conditions. However, these systems are not redundant and upon persistent loss, compensation is no longer possible.

For example, CMA is upregulated in cells of Huntington's disease patients to compensate for macroautophagy malfunctioning. However, this continuous overloading of CMA accelerates the normally occurring decline of CMA with age and contributes to accumulation of pathogenic huntingtin and other prone-to-aggregate proteins

## Why does autophagy matter?

Clearing away damaged parts is essential for keeping cells healthy and in good working order.

If junk builds up in the cell, it can permanently tweak the cell's genes, making it difficult or impossible for the cell to repair itself and regrow the structures it needs to survive and thrive.

While some cells only last in your body for a few days, others are with you for a lifetime.

Two especially important types of cells don't turn over much and are with us for decades, so it's important that they stay healthy: neurons (which are in our brains and other parts of the nervous system) and cardiomyocytes (which make up our heart muscle).

## Is Autophagy Good Or Bad For Your Health?

It's definitely good! It's also referred to as "self-devouring." While that may sound like something you never want to happen to your body, it's actually beneficial to your overall health.

This is because autophagy is an evolutionary self-preservation mechanism through which the body can remove the dysfunctional cells and recycle parts of them toward cellular repair and cleaning. "It is recycling and cleaning at the same time, just like hitting a reset button to your body. Plus, it promotes survival and adaptation as a response to various stressors and toxins accumulated in our cells. The purpose of autophagy is to remove debris and self-regulate back to optimal smooth function.

**How Autophagy Works**

It is a biological process, where the key players are tiny cells called lysosomes, which contain enzymes needed to digest and breakdown parts of the cell that no longer function properly.

That said, there is a dangerous side because lysosomes are very effective and a prolonged state of autophagy can lead to cell death, a process called autolysis. So a certain amount of autophagy is good, but too much can be damaging for our health.

**Why This Cellular Junk Removal Process Is So Necessary**

Our body needs to regularly clean out any junk that is lying around in our cells, or else our cells become less efficient and deteriorate. When our cells are not working properly, our body becomes more sensible to degeneration.

Autophagy makes our bodies more efficient, stops cancerous growth and metabolic dysfunction like diabetes and obesity.

**How Autophagy Affects Our Cells**

With it we keep our cells healthy. Our cells need cleaning from ineffective parts to avoid an imbalance between free radical damage and the antioxidants needed to prevent it. Without it, our body will experience inflammation caused by an oxidative stress.

It is also necessary to keep muscle strength as you age. By removing cellular junk your muscle stem cells continue to repair your tissues. This is the main reason detox is so important for older athletes.

## Mechanical Stress and Autophagy

When autophagy is acting as a pro-survival mechanism primarily induced by stress, it can be naturally regulated by mechanical stresses such as compression, stretching or shear stress due to fluid flow. Consistent with this, a number of studies have highlighted how cells respond to mechanical stresses by regulating autophagy levels and how this could have implications in both physiological as well as pathophysiological conditions. For instance, in response to a mechanical stimulus such as exercise, the mineralization capacity of mechano-sensitive osteoblasts is stimulated, leading to enhanced bone formation and remodeling. In relation to this, recent studies on UMR-106 rat osteoblast cell line have shown an increase in autophagy during mineralization and suggested a link between low bone density and deficiency of the autophagy protein Atg5. Such studies are indicative of the role of autophagy in regulating bone remodeling in response to mechanical stimuli.

Another recent study has demonstrated that cells induce autophagy in response to compressive stresses. Following application of compressive forces of up to 1kPa, which is within the range of normal physiological forces experienced by cells, there was a transient increase in the rate of autophagosome formation. This transient increase was suggested to function as a cellular stress management system until the cell is able to adapt to physical changes in their environment. On the other hand, excessive mechanical stresses can have an opposite effect, leading to suppression of autophagy. In a recent study, human and mouse cartilage explants subjected to high impact mechanical injuries underwent cell death, which was associated with a significant decrease in expression of autophagy markers. Interestingly, pharmacological stimulation of autophagy by rapamycin protected against cell death, highlighting the interaction between autophagy and mechanical stress in maintaining healthy cells.

**Autophagy in Cell Death**

There are three types of cell death based on the role and location of lysosomes inside the cell. Type II, later called autophagic cell death, is distinguished from type I (apoptotic) cell death by the presence of abundant autophagic structures in the dying cell, a lack of phagocyte recruitment, and, in some instances, by caspase-independence. The functional contribution of autophagy to cell death has been a subject of great controversy. The reason for controversy appears to be related to the historical focus on autophagy as a cell survival process that is described above. In addition, until relatively recently limited empirical studies had been done to test whether autophagy genes actually facilitate cell death.

Multiple experimental systems have contributed to the recent understanding of autophagy and cell death. Dictyostelium discoideum, for example, lacks apoptosis machinery that could participate in nonapoptotic cell death making this a simpler system for the interpretation of the role of autophagy in cell death. Dictyostelium exists as a unicellular organism when it is grown on rich media. Upon starvation, however, thousands of cells aggregate to form a multicellular fruiting body in which stalks support balls of spores. These stalk cells undergo developmental cell death via autophagy, as mutations in Atg genes prevent the death of stalk cells. One limitation of this system is that Dictyostelium lacks apoptosis machinery, and an understanding of the relationship between autophagy and cell death in a system with intact apoptosis machinery is important to our understanding of how to modulate autophagy for therapeutic purposes in humans.

The contribution of autophagy to cell death has been studied most in Drosophila in which apoptosis machinery is involved in the death of multiple cell types. In Drosophila, an increase in a steroid hormone triggers the destruction of obsolete tissues at the end of larval development. Dying larval midgut and salivary gland cells display markers of apoptosis, such as DNA fragmentation, acridine orange staining, and elevated levels of proapoptotic gene RNAs. These cells also possess large numbers of autophagosomes and elevated levels of Atg RNAs. Surprisingly, midgut degradation is neither disrupted by expression of the pan-caspase inhibitor p35 nor by mutation of multiple caspases, indicating that apoptosis is dispensable for developmental midgut degradatio. Interestingly, midgut destruction is blocked in animals with impaired Atg1, Atg2, or Atg18 function, directly implicating autophagy as a crucial process in steroid-induced degradation of midgut cells. Caspase deficiency does not enhance the Atg mutant midgut phenotypes, indicating that autophagic cell death in the midgut is caspase-independent.

In contrast to the Drosophila midgut, destruction of larval salivary glands requires both caspases and autophagy. Mutations in either Atg8 or Atg18 in addition to decreased function of a number of other Atg genes, all lead to the incomplete degradation of larval salivary glands. Similarly, Atg genes are required for cell death in the Drosophila amnioserosa and ovarian tissue. It is important to note that the roles and relationship of autophagy and caspases in dying salivary gland, amnioserosa, and ovarian cells in flies is cell context-specific. In addition, although larval salivary gland cell death requires both caspases and autophagy for completion of cell clearance, Atg1-induced autophagy in salivary glands is sufficient to induce premature cell death in a caspase-independent manner. Atg1 overexpression is also sufficient to cause cell death in the fat body and imaginal discs, but this death depends on caspase activity.

Studies in the nematode C. elegans also indicate that autophagy contributes to cell death. gbp-2 mutants show hyperactive muscarinic acetylcholine signaling in the pharyngeal muscle, are sensitive to starvation, and induce excess autophagy and cell death. This phenotype can be partially suppressed by either beclin-1 or Atg-7 RNAi indicating that autophagy contributes to cell death.

Autophagy is also observed in dying cells throughout mammalian development, including the regression of the corpus luteum, the involution of mammary and prostate gland and the regression of Mullerian duct structures during male genital development. Studies of derived mammalian cell lines have shown that Atg genes are required for cell death that occurs in the absence of caspase activity, but no studies to date have shown that autophagy is required for the death of mammalian cells in vivo. However, studies of beclin1 mutant murine ES cells that form embroid bodies indicates that autophagy is required for lipid signaling that is required for clearance of dying cells

# CHAPTER TWO
## THE RELATIONSHIP BETWEEN AUTOPHAGY AND APOPTOSIS

### What is Apoptosis?

Apoptosis is the process by which cells actively end their lives and is essential for maintaining cellular homeostasis. Apoptosis can be activated by a variety of cellular signals, including increased intracellular $Ca2+$ concentration, reactive oxygen species (ROS) such as hydroxyl radicals caused by oxidative damage, toxins, NO, growth factors, and hormonal stimulation. The main signaling pathway of apoptosis is the mitochondrial pathway and the death receptor pathway. Intracellular apoptosis signals usually activate the mitochondrial pathway, stimulate the activation of BH3-only protein to bind to apoptotic proteins such as Bcl-2, activate Bax/Bak aggregation to the mitochondrial membrane, and release mitochondrial pro-apoptotic proteins including cytochrome C, SMAC/DIABLO. And apoptosis-inducing factor (AIF), etc., activate the caspase cascade and induce apoptosis.

## Autophagy and Apoptosis in Cell Death

Cell death can be divided into two types, apoptosis and necrosis. Apoptosis, the first genetically programmed death process identified, is a cellintrinsic mechanism for suicide that is regulated by a variety of cellular signaling pathways. Actually, apoptosis does not determine a cell's fate alone. Autophagy, also known as type II programmed cell death, a process in which denovo-formed membrane-enclosed vesicles engulf and consume cellular components, has been shown to engage in a complex interplay with apoptosis. On one hand, it can serve as a cell survival pathway by suppressing apoptosis, for example, the removal of damaged organelles that are a source of genotoxic ROS, or by catabolizing cellular macromolecules to provide a source of nutrients and energy for the starved cell, or by limiting ER stress through the degradation of unfolded protein aggregates. On another hand, it can lead to death itself, either in collaboration with apoptosis or as a back-up mechanism when the former is defective. There are three different types of interaction between autophagy and apoptosis. Among of them, the first one type is to induce cell death in a coordinated or cooperative manner as partners; the second one is that autophagy acts as an antagonist to block apoptotic cell death by promoting cell survival; the third one is that autophagy acts as enabler of apoptosis, participating in certain morphologic and cellular events that occur during apoptotic cell death, without leading to death in itself.

## They are Partners

Numerous studies show that the mode of cooperation between autophagy and apoptosis. In this case, both autophagy and apoptosis are regulated to promote cell death. There are three types of cooperation:

(1) each of them triggers cell death synchronously;

(2) one is dominant and the other is supplemented;

(3) under circumstance of one functional defect, the other substitutes to induce cell death.

Many apoptosis-inducing stimuli often induce autophagy, for instance, both apoptosis and autophagy are simultaneously upregulated by treatment in breast cancer cells with ceramide.

Specific knockout of the autophagy-associated protein ATG7 or autophagy inhibitor 3-methyladenine inhibits caspase activation and reduces apoptosis; in many cases, the potential for autophagy-induced cell death is apoptotic Inhibition, but it plays a key role in the defect of apoptotic function. Treated Bax-/-/Bak-/- mouse embryonic fibroblasts cells with etoposide and toxic carrot lactone up-regulated cell autophagy. In these cases, autophagy and apoptosis together trigger cell death through a synergistic, complementary, or alternative mechanism.

## They are Opponents

In the confrontational relationship, autophagy runs counter to the goals and processes of apoptosis. Autophagy does not trigger cell death, but instead promotes cell survival. In endoplasmic reticulum stress, autophagy maintains endoplasmic reticulum function by digesting protein aggregates and misfolded proteins, limiting apoptosis induced by endoplasmic reticulum stress. In the cellular energy crisis, autophagy also provides energy and nutrients to cells through the digestion of large molecules such as organelles and proteins, prolonging cell life. Thus, autophagy is required for cell survival in the starvation phase of adult mice, the feeding adaptation period after sucking rats, and the nutrient-deprived cells. Autophagy is also an important mechanism for maintaining gene integrity when cells are exposed to metabolic stress, drug therapy, and radiation damage. Therefore, inhibition of autophagy in breast cancer, prostate cancer and colon cancer cells can increase the sensitivity of tumor cells to radiotherapy and chemotherapy. Mitochondrial autophagy is a kind of autophagy, which can reduce the reactive oxygen species by eliminating depolarized mitochondria and achieve the purpose of cell protection. Mitochondrial autophagy can even prevent apoptosis by reducing mitochondrial outer membrane permeabilization (MOMP) and reducing the release of mitochondrial pro-apoptotic proteins such as cytochrome C and SMAC/DIABLO.

## Autophagy is An Enabler for Apoptosis

Promoting autophagy in the relationship is not directly involved in inducing cell death, but as an energy provider to ensure that apoptosis proceeds smoothly. For example, in the case of nutrient deficiency, cells maintain intracellular ATP levels by up-regulating autophagy, allowing intracellular phosphatidylserine to release apoptosis signals to extracellular exposure. The membrane vesicle formation process of apoptotic bodies is dependent on ATP-driven actomyosin contraction. If inhibition of autophagy prevents these ATP-dependent apoptotic features, it has no effect on other apoptotic responses.

# CHAPTER THREE
## THE BENEFITS OF AUTOPHAGY

The main benefits of autophagy seem to come in the form of anti-aging principles. In fact, it's best known as the body's way of turning the clock back and creating younger cells.

Khorana points out that when our cells are stressed, autophagy is increased in order to protect us, which helps enhance your lifespan. Additionally,in times of starvation, autophagy keeps the body going by breaking down cellular material and reusing it for necessary processes.

Of course this takes energy and cannot continue forever, but it gives us more time to find nourishment. At the cellular level, the benefits of autophagy include:

**Autophagy enhances metabolic efficiency.** From the deepest cellular level, autophagy can be activated to help improve the work of the mitochondria—the cell's power plant. This makes cells work more efficiently. By doing so, autophagy helps cells become more resilient.

**Autophagy prevents neurodegenerative disorders.** Many neurodegenerative disorders are the result of damaged proteins that form in and around neurons. Autophagy protects us by getting rid of these proteins. In Huntington's disease, Parkinson's, and Alzheimer's, autophagy cleans up specific proteins associated with those diseases.

**Autophagy helps fight against infectious diseases.** It does this by removing toxins that create infection, as well as by helping to improve how your body's immune system responds to infections. Intracellular bacteria and viruses can be removed by autophagy.

**Autophagy improves muscle performance.** When exercising, we place a stress on our cells, energy goes up, and parts get worn out faster. Because of this, autophagy helps remove some of the damage and keep our energy needs in check.

Autophagy is increased in response to this in order to:

- maintain energy use balance within the cell

- reduce the amount of external energy required (by more efficiently recycling existing energy molecules)

- ensure that degraded cellular components are removed before they begin to cause any trouble

**Autophagy aids in the prevention of cancer growth.** Autophagy suppresses systems and processes that can be related to the development of cancer, such as chronic inflammation and damaged DNA. Mice altered to have inefficient autophagy were found to have higher cancer rates.

## Helps to Regulate Inflammation

Autophagy can both increase and decrease inflammation responses within the body. It increases inflammation by presenting evidence of pathogen invasion and turning on the immune response.

Autophagy then decreases the inflammation brought about by an immune response by clearing the cell of antigens that are stimulating the response. Additionally, autophagy also removes pro-immune response molecules produced by the cell in response to an invasion

## OTHER BENEFITS

- **Providing cells with molecular building blocks and energy**

- **Recycling damaged proteins, organelles and aggregates**

- **Regulating functions of cells' mitochondria,**

which help produce energy but can be damaged by oxidative stress

- Clearing damaged endoplasmic reticulum and peroxisomes

- Protecting the nervous system and encouraging growth of brain and nerve cells. Autophagy seems to improve cognitive function, brain structure and neuroplasticity.

- Supporting growth of heart cells and protecting against heart disease

- Enhancing the immune system by eliminating intracellular pathogens

- Defending against misfolded, toxic proteins that contribute to a number of amyloid diseases

- Protecting stability of DNA

- Preventing damage to healthy tissues and organs (known as necrosis)

- Potentially fighting cancer, neurodegenerative disease and other illnesses

- removing toxic proteins from the cells that are attributed to neurodegenerative diseases, such as Parkinson's and Alzheimer's disease

Autophagy is receiving a lot of attention for the role it may play in preventing or treating cancer, too. "Autophagy declines as we age, so this means cells that no longer work or may do harm are allowed to multiply, which is the MO of cancer cells."

While all cancers start from some sort of defective cells,that the body should recognize and remove those cells, often using autophagic processes. That's why some researchers are looking at the possibility that autophagy may lower the risk of cancer.

While there's no scientific evidence to back this up, some studiesTrusted Source suggest that many cancerous cells can be removed through autophagy.

"This is how the body polices the cancer villains." "Recognizing and destroying what went wrong and triggering the repairing mechanism does contribute to lowering the risk of cancer."

Researchers believe that new studies will lead to insight that will help them target autophagy as a therapy for cancer

# CHAPTER FOUR
## ACTIVATING AUTOPHAGY

There are several ways you can turn up your body's autophagy process (that have nothing to do with juice cleanses). To cleanse your cells and reduce inflammation, and generally keep your body running in tip-top shape,take these simple steps to increase the autophagy process. Keep in mind that because autophagy is a response to stress, you need to trick your body into thinking it's a little bit under siege. Certain techniques can help to optimize autophagy, and they're easy to integrate into your daily routine. Here's how:

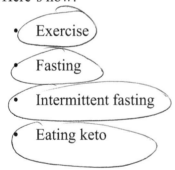

- Exercise
- Fasting
- Intermittent fasting
- Eating keto

## EXERCISE

Exercise induces autophagy in skeletal muscle in humans and the level of autophagy is affected by the intensity, duration, and modality of the exercise protocols. Several signaling pathways that are stimulated by physical exercise regulate the induction of autophagy in skeletal muscle.

Exercise, "can induce tissue recycling and regeneration in muscles, the liver, pancreas and fat tissue." Remember, autophagy is a bodily response to stress, and high-intensity exercise puts you in the good-stress sweet spot because it stresses you just enough to provoke biochemical change.

Exercise puts stress on your body. Working out actually damages your muscles, causing microscopic tears that your body then rushes to heal. This makes your muscles stronger and more resistant to any further "damage" you might cause them.

Regular exercise is the most popular way people unintentionally help their bodies cleanse themselves. (So there's actually something to that fresh, renewed feeling you get after working out.)

A 2012 study looked at autophagosomes, structures that form around pieces of cells the body has decided to recycle. After engineering mice to have glowing green autophagosomes (as one does), scientists found something interesting. The rate at which the mice were healthily demolishing their own cells drastically increased after they ran for 30 minutes on a treadmill. The rate continued to increase until the little guys had been running for 80 minutes. So, what about humans?

It's hard to figure out the amount of exercise required to switch on the autophagy boost.

"[These] are hard questions to answer at the moment," says Daniel Klionsky, PhD, a cellular biologist at the University of Michigan who specializes in autophagy. "Clearly exercise has many benefits, aside from the possible role of autophagy."

You'll get just enough impact load to make your muscles stronger (and induce autophagy) without harm. Aim for approximately 20-30 minutes a day to give your longevity an optimal boost. This points to a study from Nature showing that just 30 minutes of exercise can activate autophagy processes, so getting moving, especially in tandem with other techniques, can be a great way to activate autophagy.

Here are a few ways exercise fits in with autophagy.

• Exercise induces autophagy in peripheral tissues and in the brain. Lab mice who are defective in exercise- and starvation induced autophagy but not basal autophagy can't run as long on a treadmill as wild-type mice and don't gain the benefits of increased glucose uptake by muscle. It may even be that the growth of new brain cells by exercise is supported by autophagy.

• Exercise restores failing autophagy in damage heart tissue. Autophagy mainly targets dysfunctional mitochondria that cause inflammation and oxidative stress. There are a lot of mitochondria in the heart, liver, brain, and other vital organs. Exercise helps to eliminate these dysfunctional mitochondria thanks to autophagy.

- Autophagy promotes aerobic performance during high altitude training. Hypoxia can also stimulate autophagy and increase blood flow.

- Exercise activates the AMPK pathway, which stimulates autophagy. To activate autophagy during exercise, the activation of AMPK is also needed. AMPK regulates both protein synthesis and breakdown pathways. AMPK has a vital role in skeletal muscle homeostasis.

In addition, AMPK has been recently showed to be a critical regulator of skeletal muscle protein turnove. Protein turnover is the balance between protein build up and protein breakdown over the course of the day. If your protein synthesis exceeds the amount protein's being broken down, then you're in a more anabolic state.

## FASTING

First of all, fasting is not starvation. Starvation is the involuntary abstinence from eating forced upon by outside forces; this happens in times of war and famine when food is scarce. Fasting, on the other hand, is voluntary, deliberate, and controlled. Food is readily available but we choose not to eat it due to spiritual, health, or other reasons.

Fasting is as old as mankind, far older than any other forms of diets. Ancient civilizations, like the Greeks, recognized that there was something intrinsically beneficial to periodic fasting. They were often called times of healing, cleansing, purification, or detoxification. Virtually every culture and religion on earth practice some rituals of fasting.

Before the advent of agriculture, humans never ate three meals a day plus snacking in between. We ate only when we found food which could be hours or days apart. Hence, from an evolution standpoint, eating three meals a day is not a requirement for survival. Otherwise, we would not have survived as a species.

Fast forward to the 21st century, we have all forgotten about this ancient practice. After all, fasting is really bad for business! Food manufacturers encourage us to eat multiple meals and snacks a day. Nutritional authorities warn that skipping a single meal will have dire health consequences. Overtime, these messages have been so well-drilled into our heads.

Fasting has no standard duration. It may be done for a

few hours to many days to months on end. Fasting is the "safest and best-proven strategy" for triggering autophagy, Fasting is our "evolutionary trigger" for stimulating this natural process.

"Eating inhibits autophagy by switching on the enzyme called mTOR, which is a powerful inhibitor of autophagy." Fasting, on the contrary, allows this enzyme to switch off, thus stimulating autophagy.

There are a number of different ways to integrate the benefits of fasting into your daily life, starting with a simple slight lowering of caloric intake and ranging to full, multi-day fasts. While studies suggest that a 24- to 48-hour fast is ideal for the stimulation of autophagy, a 12-hour fast is a good start – and that's something you can do fairly easily by abstaining from eating for a few hours before going to bed.

## What Happens When We Fast?

The process of using and storing food energy that occurs when we eat goes in reverse when we fast. Insulin levels drop, prompting the body to start burning stored energy. Glycogen, the glucose that is stored in the liver, is first accessed and used. After that, the body starts to break down stored body fat for energy.

Thus, the body basically exists in two states - the fed state with high insulin and the fasting state with low insulin. We are either storing food energy or we are burning food energy. If eating and fasting are balanced, then there is no weight gain. If we spend the majority of the day eating and storing energy, there is a good chance that overtime we may end up gaining weight.

## INTERMITTENT FASTING (IF)

Fasting, or periods of voluntary abstinence from food has been practiced throughout the world for ages. Intermittent Fasting refers to dietary eating patterns that involve not eating or severely restricting calories for a prolonged period of time. Intermittent fasting is an eating pattern where we cycle between fasting and regular eating. Shorter fasts of 16-20 hours are generally done more frequently, even daily. Longer fasts, typically 24-36 hours, are done 2-3 times per week. As it happens, we all fast daily for a period of 12 hours or so between dinner and breakfast. There are many different subgroups of intermittent fasting each with individual variation in the duration of the fast; some for hours, others for day(s). This has become an extremely popular topic in the science community due to all of the potential benefits on fitness and health that are being discovered.

Intermittent fasting with the goal of improving health relatively new. Intermittent fasting involves restricting intake of food for a set period of time and does not include any changes to the actual foods you are eating. Currently, the most common Intermittent fasting protocols are a daily 16 hour fast and fasting for a whole day, one or two days per week. Intermittent fasting could be considered a natural eating pattern that humans are built to implement and it traces all the way back to our paleolithic hunter-gatherer ancestors. The current model of a planned program of intermittent fasting could potentially help improve many aspects of health from body composition to longevity and aging. Although Intermittent fasting goes against the norms of our culture and common daily routine, the science may be pointing to less meal frequency and more time fasting as the optimal alternative to the normal breakfast, lunch, and dinner model.

Intermittent fasting isn't just a weight loss strategy or a hack that bodybuilders use to lose fat quickly while maintaining lean muscle mass. It is at its best a healthy lifestyle informed by human evolution and the study of metabolism. It asks the human body to be much more efficient and self-protective than it is accustomed to being in modern times.

There are many things that happen when we fast that either don't happen when we are always in a fed state, or that happen very slowly in the background of glucose metabolism.

In a well-fed state, the individual cell in your body is in "growth" mode. Its insulin signaling and mTOR pathways that tell the cell to grow, divide and synthesize proteins are active. By the way, these pathways, when overactive, have implications in cancer growth.

By skipping breakfast and eating all of your meals within an eight-hour window, you will increase your body's inherent autophagy process. Like a protein-specific fast, intermittent fasting gives your body a chance to "catch up" on all those lingering toxins by cleaning up in real-time. Remove toxin build-up with a 16-28 hour fast. If done incorrectly, intermittent fasting can cause hormone imbalances in women. That's because women are highly sensitive to signs of starvation or calorie restriction. To sidestep issues, consume a fat-only breakfast, like Bulletproof Coffee.

"When you are intermittent fasting, "you are literally telling every cell in your body to activate autophagy and to clean out the cells."

## METHODS OF INTERMITTENT FASTING:

Intermittent fasting comes in various forms and each may have a specific set of unique benefits. Each form of intermittent fasting has variations in the fasting-to-eating ratio. The benefits and effectiveness of these different protocols may differ on an individual basis and it is important to determine which one is best for you. Factors that may influence which one to choose include health goals, daily schedule/routine, and current health status. The most common types of IF are alternate day fasting, time-restricted feeding, and modified fasting.

### Alternate Day Fasting:

This approach involves alternating days of absolutely no calories (from food or beverage) with days of free feeding and eating whatever you want.

This plan has been shown to help with weight loss, improve blood cholesterol and triglyceride (fat) levels, and improve markers for inflammation in the blood.

The main downfall with this form of intermittent fasting is that it is the most difficult to stick with because of the reported hunger during fasting days.

**Modified Fasting - 5:2 Diet**

Modified fasting is a protocol with programmed fasting days, but the fasting days do allow for some food intake. Generally 20-25% of normal calories are allowed to be consumed on fasting days; so if you normally consume 2000 calories on regular eating days, you would be allowed 400-500 calories on fasting days. The 5:2 part of this diet refers to the ratio of non-fasting to fasting days. So on this regimen you would eat normally for 5 consecutive days, then fast or restrict calories to 20-25% for 2 consecutive days.

This protocol is great for weight loss, body composition, and may also benefit the regulation of blood sugar, lipids, and inflammation. Studies have shown the 5:2 protocol to be effective for weight loss, improve/lower inflammation markers in the blood (3), and show signs trending improvements in insulin resistance. In animal studies, this modified fasting 5:2 diet resulted in decreased fat, decreased hunger hormones (leptin), and increased levels of a protein responsible for improvements in fat burning and blood sugar regulation (adiponectin).

The modified 5:2 fasting protocol is easy to follow and has a small number of negative side effects which included hunger, low energy, and some irritability when beginning the program. Contrary to this however, studies have also noted improvements such as reduced tension, less anger, less fatigue, improvements in self confidence, and a more positive mood.

## Time-Restricted Feeding:

If you know anyone that has said they are doing intermittent fasting, odds are it is in the form of time-restricted feeding. This is a type of intermittent fasting that is used daily and it involves only consuming calories during a small portion of the day and fasting for the remainder. Daily fasting intervals in time-restricted feeding may range from 12-20 hours, with the most common method being 16/8 (fasting for 16 hours, consuming calories for 8). For this protocol the time of day is not important as long as you are fasting for a consecutive period of time and only eating in your allowed time period. For example, on a 16/8 time-restricted feeding program one person may eat their first meal at 7AM and last meal at 3PM (fast from 3PM-7AM), while another person may eat their first meal at 1PM and last meal at 9PM (fast from 9PM-1PM). This protocol is meant to be performed every day over long periods of time and is very flexible as long as you are staying within the fasting/eating window(s).

Time-Restricted feeding is one of the most easy to follow methods of intermittent fasting. Using this along with your daily work and sleep schedule may help achieve optimal metabolic function. Time-restricted feeding is a great program to follow for weight loss and body composition improvements as well as some other overall health benefits. The few human trials that were conducted noted significant reductions in weight, reductions in fasting blood glucose, and improvements in cholesterol with no changes in perceived tension, depression, anger, fatigue, or confusion. Some other preliminary results from animal studies showed time restricted feeding to protect against obesity, high insulin levels, fatty liver disease, and inflammation.

The easy application and promising results of time-restricted feeding could possibly make it an excellent option for weight loss and chronic disease prevention/management. When implementing this protocol it may be good to begin with a lower fasting-to-eating ratio like 12/12 hours and eventually work your way up to 16/8 hours

## Intermittent Fasting Versus Continuous Calorie-Restriction

The portion-control strategy of constant caloric reduction is the most common dietary recommendation for weight loss and type 2 diabetes. For example, the American Diabetes Association recommends a 500-750 kcal/day energy deficit coupled with regular physical activity. Dietitians follow this approach and recommend eating 4-6 small meals throughout the day.

Does the portion-control strategy work in the long-run? Rarely. A cohort study with a 9-year follow-up from the United Kingdom on 176,495 obese individuals indicated that only 3,528 of them succeeded in attaining normal body weight by the end of the study. That is a failure rate of 98%! Intermittent fasting is not constant caloric restriction. Restricting calories causes a compensatory increase in hunger and worse, a decrease in the body's metabolic rate, a double curse! Because when we are burning fewer calories per day, it becomes increasingly harder to lose weight and much easier to gain weight back after we have lost it. This type of diet puts the body into a "starvation mode" as metabolism revs down to conserve energy. Intermittent fasting does not have any of these drawbacks.

## INTERMITTENT FASTING FOR WOMEN

For women who are interested in weight loss, intermittent fasting may seem like a great choice, but many people want to know, should women fast? Is intermittent fasting effective for women? There have been a few key studies about intermittent fasting which can help to shed some light on this interesting new dietary trend.

Intermittent fasting is also known as alternate-day fasting, although there are certainly some variations on this diet. The American Journal of Clinical Nutrition performed a study that enrolled 16 obese men and women on a 10-week program. On the fasting days, participants consumed food to 25% of their estimated energy needs. The rest of the time, they received dietary counseling, but were not given a specific guideline to follow during this time.

As expected, the participants lost weight due to this study, but what researchers really found interesting were some specific changes. The subjects were all still obese after just 10 weeks, but they had shown improvement in cholesterol, LDL-cholesterol, triglycerides, and systolic blood pressure. What made this an interesting find was that most people have to lose more weight than these study participants before seeing the same changes. It was a fascinating find which has spurred a great number of people to try fasting.

Intermittent fasting for women has some beneficial effects. What makes it especially important for women who are trying to lose weight is that women have a much higher fat proportion in their bodies. When trying to lose weight, the body primarily burns through carbohydrate stores with the first 6 hours and then starts to burn fat. Women who are following a healthy diet and exercise plan may be struggling with stubborn fat, but fasting is a realistic solution to this.

## INTERMITTENT FASTING FOR WOMEN OVER 50

Obviously our bodies and our metabolism changes when we hit menopause. One of the biggest changes that women over 50 experience is that they have a slower metabolism and they start to put on weight. Fasting may be a good way to reverse and prevent this weight gain though. Studies have shown that this fasting pattern helps to regulate appetite and people who follow it regularly do not experience the same cravings that others do. If you're over 50 and trying to adjust to your slower metabolism, intermittent fasting can help you to avoid eating too much on a daily basis.

When you reach 50, your body also starts to develop some chronic diseases like high cholesterol and high blood pressure. Intermittent fasting has been shown to decrease both cholesterol and blood pressure, even without a great deal of weight loss. If you've started to notice your numbers rising at the doctor's office each year, you may be able to bring them back down with fasting, even without losing much weight. Intermittent fasting may not be a great idea for every woman.

## HEALTH BENEFITS OF INTERMITTENT FASTING

Research on intermittent fasting is in it's infancy but it still has huge potential for weight loss and the treatment of some chronic disease. Here are the possible benefits of intermittent fasting:

### Increases metabolism leading to weight and body fat loss

Unlike a daily caloric reduction diet, intermittent fasting raises metabolism. This makes sense from a survival standpoint. If we do not eat, the body uses stored energy as fuel so that we can stay alive to find another meal. Hormones allow the body to switch energy sources from food to body fat.

Studies demonstrate this phenomenon clearly. For example, four days of continuous fasting increased Basal Metabolic Rate by 12%. Levels of the neurotransmitter norepinephrine, which prepares the body for action, increased by 117%. Fatty acids in the bloodstream increased over 370% as the body switched from burning food to burning stored fats.

### No loss in muscle mass

Unlike a constant calorie-restriction diet, intermittent

fasting does not burn muscles as many have feared. In 2010, researchers looked at a group of subjects who underwent 70 days of alternate daily fasting (ate one day and fasted the next). Their muscle mass started off at 52.0 kg and ended at 51.9 kg. In other words, there was no loss of muscles but they did lose 11.4% of fat and saw major improvements in LDL cholesterol and triglyceride levels.

During fasting, the body naturally produces more human growth hormone to preserve lean muscles and bones. Muscle mass is generally preserved until body fat drops below 4%. Therefore, most people are not at risk of muscle-wasting when doing intermittent fasting.

## Reverses insulin resistance, type 2 diabetes, and fatty liver

Type 2 diabetes is a condition whereby there is simply too much sugar in the body, to the point that the cells can no longer respond to insulin and take in any more glucose from the blood (insulin resistance), resulting in high blood sugar. Also, the liver becomes loaded with fat as it tries to clear out the excess glucose by converting it to and storing it as fat.

Therefore, to reverse this condition, two things have to happen -

- First, stop putting more sugar into the body.

- Second, burn the remaining sugar off.

The best diet to achieve this is a low-carbohydrate, moderate-protein, and high-healthy fat diet, also called ketogentic diet. (Remember that carbohydrate raises blood sugar the most, protein to some degree, and fat the least.) That is why a low-carb diet will help reduce the burden of incoming glucose. For some people, this is already enough to reverse insulin resistance and type 2 diabetes. However, in more severe cases, diet alone is not sufficient.

What about exercise? Exercise will help burn off glucose in the skeletal muscles but not all the tissues and organs, including the fatty liver. Clearly, exercise is important, but to eliminate the excess glucose in the organs, there is the need to temporarily "starve" the cells.

Intermittent fasting can accomplish this. That is why historically, people called fasting a cleanse or a detox. It can be a very powerful tool to get rid of all the excesses. It is the fastest way to lower blood glucose and insulin levels, and eventually reversing insulin resistance, type 2 diabetes, and fatty liver.

By the way, taking insulin for type 2 diabetes does not address the root cause of the problem, which is excess sugar in the body. It is true that insulin will drive the glucose away from the blood, resulting in lower blood glucose, but where does the sugar go? The liver is just going to turn it all into fat, fat in the liver and fat in the abdomen. Patients who go on insulin often end up gaining more weight, which worsens their diabetes.

**Enhances heart health**

Overtime, high blood glucose from type 2 diabetes can damage the blood vessels and nerves that control the heart. The longer one has diabetes, the higher the chances that heart disease will develop. By lowering blood sugar through intermittent fasting, the risk of cardiovascular disease and stroke is also reduced.

In addition, intermittent fasting has been shown to improve blood pressure, total and LDL (bad) cholesterol, blood triglycerides, and inflammatory markers associated with many chronic diseases.

**Boosts brain power**

Multiple studies demonstrated fasting has many neurologic benefits including attention and focus, reaction time, immediate memory, cognition, and generation of new brain cells. Mice studies also showed that intermittent fasting reduces brain inflammation and prevents the symptoms of Alzheimer's.

## INTERMITTENR FASTING SHOWN IN ANIMAL STUDIES:

1. Decreased Body Fat

2. Decreased levels of the hunger hormone leptin

3. Improve insulin levels

4. Protect against obesity, fatty liver disease, and inflammation

5. Longevity

## HOW INTERMITTENT FASTING AFFECTS YOUR CELLS AND HORMONES

When you fast, several things happen in your body on the cellular and molecular level. For example, your body adjusts hormone levels to make stored body fat more accessible. Your cells also initiate important repair processes and change the expression of genes.

Here are some changes that occur in your body when you fast:

- Human Growth Hormone (HGH): The levels of growth hormone skyrocket, increasing as much as 5-fold. This has benefits for fat loss and muscle gain, to name a few.

- Insulin: Insulin sensitivity improves and levels of insulin drop dramatically. Lower insulin levels make stored body fat more accessible.

- Cellular repair: When fasted, your cells initiate cellular repair processes. This includes autophagy, where cells digest and remove old and dysfunctional proteins that build up inside cells

- Gene expression: There are changes in the function of genes related to longevity and protection against disease.

These changes in hormone levels, cell function and gene expression are responsible for the health benefits of intermittent fasting.

## WHAT TO EXPECT WITH INTERMITTENT FASTING

### Hunger Goes Down

We normally feel hunger pangs about four hours after a meal. So if we fast for 24 hours, does it mean that our hunger sensations will be six times more severe? Of course not.

Many people are concerned that fasting will result in extreme hunger and overeating. Studies showed that on the day after a one-day fast, there is, indeed, a 20% increase in caloric intake. However, with repeated fasting, hunger and appetite surprisingly decrease.

Hunger comes in waves. If we do nothing, the hunger dissipates after a while. Drinking tea (all kinds) or coffee (with or without caffeine) is often enough to fight it off. However, it is best to drink it black though a teaspoon or two of cream or half-and-half will not trigger much insulin response. Do not use any types of sugar or artificial sweeteners. If necessary, bone broth can also be taken during fasting.

## Blood sugar does not crash

Sometimes people worry that blood sugar will fall very low during fasting and they will become shaky and sweaty. This does not actually happen as blood sugar is tightly monitored by the body and there are multiple mechanisms to keep it in the proper range. During fasting, the body begins to break down glycogen in the liver to release glucose. This happens every night during our sleep.

If we fast for longer than 24-36 hours, glycogen stores become depleted and the liver will manufacture new glucose using glycerol which is a by-product of the breakdown of fat (a process called gluconeogenesis). Apart from using glucose, our brain cells can also use ketones for energy. Ketones are produced when fat is metabolized and they can supply up to 75% of the brain's energy requirements (the other 25% from glucose).

The only exception is for those who are taking diabetic medications and insulin. You MUST first consult your doctor as the dosages will probably need to be reduced while you are fasting. Otherwise, if you overmedicate and hypoglycemia develops, which can be dangerous, you must have some sugar to reverse it. This will break the fast and make it counterproductive.

**The dawn phenomenon**

After a period of fasting, especially in the morning, some people experience high blood glucose. This dawn phenomenon is a result of the circadian rhythm whereby just before awakening, the body secretes higher levels of several hormones to prepare for the upcoming day -

- Adrenaline - to give the body some energy

- Growth hormone - to help repair and make new protein

- Glucagon - to move glucose from storage in the liver to the blood for use as energy

- Cortisol, the stress hormone - to activate the body

These hormones peak in the morning hours, then fall to lower levels during the day. In non-diabetics, the magnitude of the blood sugar rise is small and most people will not even notice it. However, for the majority of the diabetics, there can be a noticeable spike in blood glucose as the liver dumps sugar into the blood.

This will happen in extended fasts too. When there is no food, insulin levels stay low while the liver releases some of its stored sugar and fat. This is natural and not a bad thing at all. The magnitude of the spike will decrease as the liver becomes less bloated with sugar and fat.

## WHO SHOULD BE CAREFUL OR AVOID INTERMITTENT FASTING?

- Women who want to get pregnant, are pregnant, or are breastfeeding.

- Those who are malnourished or underweight.

- Children under 18 years of age and elders.

- Those who have gout.

- Those who have gastroesophageal reflux disease (GERD).

- Those who have eating disorders should first consult with their doctors.

- Those who are taking diabetic medications and insulin must first consult with their doctors as dosages will need to be reduced.

- Those who are taking medications should first consult with their doctors as the timing of medications may be affected.

- Those who feel very stressed or have cortisol issues should not fast because fasting is another stressor.

- Those who are training very hard most days of the week should not fast.

Intermittent fasting is certainly not for everyone. If you're underweight or have a history of eating disorders, you should not fast without consulting with a health professional first. JIn these cases, it can be downright harmful.

## DANGERS OF INTERMITTENT FASTING

### Nutrient Deficiencies

Any fasting protocol can put you at risk for nutrient deficiencies. By restricting calories, you are also restricting essential vitamins, minerals, fatty acids, amino acids, and electrolytes—all things your body needs to function properly.

### Dehydration

Even though you drink water during a water fast, you can be at risk for dehydration. For most people, at least 20 percent of daily water consumption comes from the foods you eat. If you don't increase your water intake during the fast, you will actually end up consuming much less water than usual.

### Hypotension

On the other hand, if you drink too much water, you may experience hypotension. Hypotension is extremely low blood pressure—the opposite of hypertension, or high blood pressure.

Additionally, you may experience orthostatic hypotension, which involves sudden drops in blood pressure upon standing up. Orthostatic hypotension can cause dizziness and lightheadedness.

## Hyponatremia

Also called water intoxication, hyponatremia occurs when the water and salt lost through sweating are replaced by water only. You shouldn't exercise during a water fast because you will lose salt through perspiration and won't be able to replace it by eating food or drinking sports beverages.

## Dizziness, Fatigue, and Trouble Focusing

Dizziness, fatigue, and brain fog are all symptoms of extreme calorie restriction. When you don't consume the number of calories your body needs, your body will struggle to perform at an optimal level. It may become difficult to focus at work or school during a water fast. Fasting can also cause mild-to-severe headaches.

## Binge Eating

Fasting—and dieting or restricting calories in general—often leads to binge eating. Fasting can also lead to obsessive or intrusive thoughts about food, which may cause you to binge eat when your water fast is over.

## EATING KETO

The high-fat ketogenic diet has become popular in many health circles for its anti-inflammatory benefits, and it's also incredibly useful for triggering autophagy. "Ketones are high in energy, potent antioxidants (so they drop inflammation dramatically), and extremely restorative to nerve cells - improving the health and function of the brain and entire nervous system."

The key, however, is to opt for a healthful ketogenic diet – which means abstaining from some of the heavier, cheese-and-bacon-based keto recipes you'll find online. Opting for a plant-heavy ketogenic diet is the healthiest approach, and keeping protein lower is also important.

Many people "misunderstand" keto, turning it into "this high-protein, high-animal-fat experience."

"But the reality is that it's truly about the good fats and getting the fats into the body at the right time as well." Consuming fat first thing in the morning, reserving any carbohydrate consumption for the end of the day, is the best way to prevent an insulin spike and support the activation of autophagy.

## Ketosis - What is It?

Ketosis is a state in metabolism when the liver converts fat into fatty acids and ketone bodies which can then be used by the body for energy. This is not to be confused with "ketoacidosis" which is a dangerous condition that can occur with diabetes. Ketosis is the state that we all want to reach to lose weight. Ketones are molecules generated by the liver during fat metabolism and are a normal source of fuel and energy for the body. Diets that restrict calorie intake cause weight loss, however, some of the weight loss is from fat and some of it is from lean muscle tissue. The loss of lean muscle tissue slows the metabolism making weight loss more difficult and also makes regaining weight easier.

When your body is in ketosis, it is using fat as its' primary source of energy. If you are consuming adequate protein, your body will not break down muscle tissue. Once your liver has converted fat into ketones, they cannot be converted back to fat and stored, so the body must excrete the molecules in your sweat and urine.

Many people falsely believe they cannot or are not losing weight because the ketones drop to a lower level. This means that Ketostiks which are used to measure the ketones in the urine, are no longer showing the purple color on the test strip, but weight loss continues with or without the ketones being present. The excess ketones excreted in the urine disappear on a low-carbohydrate diet after the body becomes accustomed to using dietary fats for energy instead of glucose. This usually occurs within a few weeks on the diet. People who normally eat high-carbohydrate meals have been fueling their bodies from the glucose and fructose obtained from the carbohydrates. Their cells have had very little experience burning fatty acids for energy. The body uses the glucose first to prevent high levels of glucose in the blood.

The body experiences a new condition when a person goes on the low-carbohydrate diet. The more commonly used glucose fuel is no longer available. The body reacts by dropping the pancreas' production of insulin and increasing the hormone glucagon. The glucagon draws stored fat reserves in the form of triglycerides for use by the cells as the new energy source. However, the cells are slow to react to this new fuel source, and the individual feels weakness or a lack of energy. The resistance to burn fatty acids for energy can vary greatly between individuals. Some people feel weak while others have a feeling of greater energy than before.

The liver begins to catabolize (break down) the extra fatty acids which are not being utilized by the cells. However, the liver does not have the enzyme necessary for complete catabolism of the fatty acids. This causes the discharge of the ketone molecules into the blood. The strange taste in the mouth and mild breath odor shows the presence of these ketones. Other body cells can utilize the ketones for energy. The brain can also utilize ketones contrary to the myth that the brain must be powered by glucose only; although, some areas of the brain still require glucose, which the body makes from amino acids or fats. The body begins to utilize the fatty acids for energy more efficiently after a few weeks and the ketone level drops to normal. This does not mean one is not losing weight. It means the body is becoming a more efficient fat burner.

# CHAPTER FIVE
## AUTOPHAGY PERFORMANCE

### Steps To Water Fasting

When you fast, the water will replenishes your body's source of vital life energy - water. Without water, the human body cannot function, repair or sustain. Drinking nothing but water renews the body's building blocks with fresh raw material (oxygen and hydrogen) to renew itself. Water fasting flushes your cells with this fresh material and forces the old toxins and chemicals into the bloodstream. There, they are detoxified by the liver, kidneys and skin.

Water fasting is considered very challenging but it can be rewarding as you would feel a total cleansed body. Once you have completed a longer fast, you can maintain your new level of health by using smaller water fasts. 1-3 days on water fast every now and then will help keep your body "in tune" and detoxified. But definitely, a proper diet and lifestyle will contribute to keeping your body free and clear of toxin accumulation.

**Step #1: Start small** - You don't know how your body will react to fasting at first, so only plan your first fast for 24-hours, which essentially means skipping a few meals and all snack.

- The right day to take up this fast would be to choose a day when you have lesser activities planned. If there are excessive activities, then they consume a lot of calories and that will make you hungry

- Fasting should ideally start in the morning by drinking about two glasses of water which will clear your bowel movement

- Simple pure water is the best. Boiled or cool water will also do. Drinking 1 ½ liters to 3 liters of plain water in one full day depending on individual capacity is good. You can drink more if you are up for it. I honestly did not count mine

- Few bodily reactions which may seem scary but are considered normal and you all will experience as well if you are water fasting for the first time. Some of the signs are weakness, dizziness and nausea and these are common due to the sudden lack of food. I personally experienced a slight drop in blood pressure and headaches during the latter part of the day. The key to this is just lie down and relax whenever these symptoms become intense. The more difficult you find it, the more it means that your body has a lot of toxins to clean out

- Towards mid-day, you will feel a sudden bout of hunger. Just have one or two glasses of water to dilute the gastric secretions. Then lie down and take rest. The hunger should go away in a short time

**Step #2: Water Only -** Drink lots of water during your fast, maybe 12 or more glasses, to make sure you stay hydrated and because your system will need the water to help flush out the toxins that will leave your body during the fast. If you can, use distilled water, which will have a better cleansing effect than tap water.

**Step #3: Get Rest -** Plan your fasting day so that you won't be doing any heavy lifting or strenuous physical tasks. Your body needs to focus on itself and you need to give it the kind of rest that will allow it to do that. Plan to get maybe an hour more sleep than you usually get. Not only will you find you'll need it, but this is also one less waking hour that you'll be thinking about how nice it would be to have something to eat!

**Step #4: Ease your way off -** When the fast period is up, don't dig into a huge meal, even if you are tempted to do so. Eat something small, and have some juice to give your body a quick shot of energy. If you don't have any pain or digestive issues, then you can work up to a larger meal later in the day.

**Step #5:** After having fasted, learning how to break a fast is important. As there is hardly any digestive activity during fasting, one should be very careful while breaking the fast. The best way to break a fast is with lime juice or orange juice which will make the stomach alkaline. It's wiser to have few spices and no oily food during this time. Second meal of the day can be normal Before you do any of this, make sure you are healthy enough to fast, and if you are in doubt, consult with your doctor.

## WEIGHT LOSS AND WATER FASTING

Attempting to lose weight is one of the biggest task you can ever get. With the list of lifestyle changes you make in order to lose weight. It is usually tedious and tiring to keep up with calories, portions, vitamins and regular exercise.

Weight loss is not as hard as many think it is but the problem is, one of the easiest way to lose weight is usually over looked. Water fasting and weight loss have a lot in good. By drinking at least 8 glasses of water per day, you can lose weight in no time and also improve your general wellness. Water works wonder in your system by acting as appetite suppressant, helping you to grow healthily and also improve your metabolic rate. The success of weight loss with water is due to it abilities to work as a appetite suppressant. You less hunger pangs whenever you drink as much as 8 glasses of water per day.

As a dieter, the more water you drink, the more the extra pounds you lose. In order to lose weight and to lose it fast, you need to burn extra fats and calories from your body, a result which dehydrates your internal body. Therefore if you don't provide your body with the needed amount of water, it may result into serious health problems such as the malfunctioning of your kidneys and liver.

You may have to visit the bathroom more due to an increase in the amount of what you take in daily but you don't have to let this stop you from drinking more water as it is what your body needs most in order to shed those extra pounds in no time. The fact that you may be visiting the bathroom more often than usual does not mean you are drinking too much water. In fact the more you visit the bathroom the better as it means something good is already happening to you. Your body is only reacting to the increase of water supply and is already flushing out toxins from your bloodstream. Once your body knows it can depend on the water being supplied to it by you, you will begin to see the swollen ankles, hips, and thighs trimming down as the excess water is flushed out. Drinking more water enhances your fat burning ability. You can lose lot of weight with regular exercise and eating habit but you still need lot and lot of water to keep your body hydrated. You must use water-included vegetables and fruits as well. Other than losing weight, drinking water has a lot of benefits like it boosts your energy levels, it helps reduce blood pressure, it helps reduce high cholesterol, and it improves your skin and increase body freshness.

Here are the main 3 intermittent fasting for weight loss benefits that stand out the most:

- **Detoxification -** It is one of the most important fasting benefits of all. As you fast, undergoes a self cleaning process, when freed from constant food processing. This allows it to wipe out your body toxins accumulated during heavy lunches or quick fast-food meals. And after that, you feel just great!

- **Developing patience -** Most people tend to overlook this enormous fasting benefit. Unfortunately, most of us actually lack this important quality, not only during diets, but mostly in everyday life. You see, patience comes from self-control, and this one is like a muscle: the more you train it, the stronger it gets. So, along with other fasting benefits, you also become stronger mentally!

- **Effective weight loss -** of course! Nowadays it's the main fasting benefit, and the key reason why most people get into it is fasting for weight loss. Actually, our bodies are designed to live long without food, as we did in the olden days. When we eat, our liver and muscles store energy as glycogen. In the fasting days, our body uses glycogen first for a couple of hours, then it starts burning off the fat.

## How does water fasting and weight loss work today?

Unlike crash diets (otherwise known as fad diets), intermittent fasting doesn't require you to go without food for days on end. It just takes advantage of that window of opportunity that comes roughly 24 hours after your last meal to help burn those calories, not to mention the money you'll save on groceries or the various health benefits that go along with it like lower blood pressure and, most important of all, effective weight loss.

While staying without food is not a sacrifice many people would be willing to make, let's just see if it's a method worth trying. First of all, many detoxification methods are very expensive and most people can barely afford them. This simple and cheap approach may even be better than the rest. This process gives the body a chance to clean and maintain itself by taking its attention off the digestion of food for sometime. This is the body's method of cleaning its own. As a matter of fact, a new cycle will kick in the body once it's done with the detoxification. This way, it would have gotten rid of all toxins that have built up in the body and the accumulating wastes too.

And so, within the first three days you may begin to notice some physiological changes. Since the body's energy source is glucose, which comes from the foods we consume, this energy is stored as glycogen in our bodies. This energy is enough to sustain the body for a day but will be exhausted faster during this fasting.

So if you are still wondering how this works in weight loss, here we go. After the body has consumed all the glycogen in the liver, it starts using the excess fat to replace the exhausted glycogen. This will normally be on the second day and the body will convert these fatty acids into glucose. Consequently, the body is taking in a lot of water and as a result the bowel too is undergoing some cleansing.

Hence in this entire process, the body organs will undergo intensive repair. The body's digestive system is given time to recover while at the same time ensuring that no toxins enter the system. But the important thing is that you will have detoxified your body and lost some weight too.

But there are several precautions that one should take while doing water fasting weight loss. While it's a good approach, we should be quite cautious in how we undertake the entire process. To start with, the best water to consume for this approach should be distilled water.

Again it requires a lot of common sense; not everyone can fast however hard they are dying to lose weight. Those with a weak metabolism may not have the ability to process the fatty acids. If you are malnourished or starving, it too will not be the best method to use. Pregnant women must never use it since the baby and the mother are in dire need of the nutrients.

So sit back in your quest to lose weight and think whether water fasting weight loss will work for you. Just because it works for others does not necessarily mean it's the best for you.

## Tips on Intermittent Fasting For Weight Loss

Intermittent fasting is without a doubt one of the fastest and most efficient ways to lose body-fat and do better. But how do you go about it? Here are 5 tips to help you get started on an effective intermittent fasting diet.

## 1. Don't make your fast too long or too short

An ideal fast length for weight-loss and health benefits is between 16 and 24 hours depending on age, experience and exact goals. Any less than this won't really give you the results you want (remember you are already fasting for 10-12 hours overnight) and any longer than this is simply unnecessary and can be harder to adapt to.

## 2. Increase your water intake when fasting

Intermittent fasting will also help to cleanse your system and let your body work more efficiently. In order to help this process, you should increase your water intake. The best way to do this is have a glass/bottle of water with you at all times so that you can sip regularly.

## 3. Break your fast with a healthy meal

The first thing you eat after a fast should be a healthy meal. Apart from the obvious benefits of eating healthy food, this also leaves less space for eating junk. Given that you might only have 8 hours to eat your daily food, filling up on the good stuff first is always a good option.

## 4. Time your food around your workouts

It goes without saying that working out should be part of any healthy eating plan. The centre piece of your training efforts should be weight-training or bodyweight training. Try to eat most of your food in the period immediately after your workout. In this way your body will be more likely to use these calories to rebuild and repair rather than be stocked as fat.

## 5. Don't Cheat

Don't fool your self by thinking if you just have a little bite it wont matter, you might just need to eat something, but by doing this your putting a pause on the fasting process.

## 6. Don't sweat the details

One of the real benefits of intermittent fasting is that it is not necessary to count calories or grams of macronutrients. This can be a pain and makes diets difficult to stick to. Follow principles and the details will take care of themselves.

## Advantages Of That Natural Weight Loss Food (Water)

**1. Fight Dehydration -** Dehydration has several subtle effects that may upset your weight loss, one of those though is that dehydration slows down the fat burning process. When your system cannot flush the toxins out of your body that are created by burning up fat, it simply can not burn them as fast. This is a preservation mechanism as you don't need to have problems with too much toxicity inside your body.

**2. Combat Injury -** Drinking plenty of water helps to make certain that the joints are completely lubricated. This helps them to perform properly and lessens the possibility of injury to the joints. Hydrating your muscles also keeps them elastic so that they'll properly flex and contract. This helps make certain that you are working at peak performance when you're exercising.

**3. Oxygenated muscles** - Certainly one of the most essential factors to getting an effective work out is making certain your muscles are appropriately oxygenated. When you're dehydrated, the volume of your blood is smaller than when you are hydrated. This smaller volume of blood means that less oxygen will get to your muscles and that they can fatigue more swiftly.

**4. Improve Recovery Time** - Subsequent to working out, you are likely to feel drained and you will often feel sore, especially the subsequent day. While many believe that this is attributable to lactic acid, it's more likely that the soreness felt is because of tissue damage. That said though, there are chemicals made if you work out and being properly hydrated can help flush those toxins out of the muscles faster than when you're dehydrated.

5. **Fight Hungry Feeling** - One of the ways in which our bodies signal that it's dehydrated is that it produces an empty feeling in our stomach. Unfortunately, we tend to usually interpret this feeling as a want for food and we eat unnecessarily. An easy means to determine if you are hungry or truly

dehydrated is to drink some water once you get that feeling and then wait roughly fifteen minutes. If you continue to feel hungry, it is time to eat. If not, you were merely thirsty

## MASS MUSCLE AND WATER FASTING

As you know, your body is constantly burning energy in the form of protein, carbohydrates and fat. When you eat food, your body is in the "fed" state and is focused on digesting the food and adding up fat stores in your body for future energy.

When your body doesn't have anything left to digest, it flips over to the "fasted" state where it starts burning off calories as well as healing your internal organs in a pretty dramatic way.

But one of the greatest thing that happens after a few hours of not having any food in your system is that your body automatically starts to increase the production of human growth hormone (HGH) - one of the most powerful anti-aging and muscle building chemicals in your body. At the end of a 24 hour period, it produces between 5-600% more human growth hormone than if you had food!

Although many people think that not eating will cause your muscles to breakdown, and to a certain extent they're right, over a 24 hour period the boost in human growth hormone counteracts the fact that there is no new protein in your body so it preserves your muscles!

Also, studies have been showing that when you do water fasting for weight loss and your HGH levels go up, you start releasing more fatty acids into your bloodstream, which is what happens as you burn fat.

Intermittent fasting and bodybuilding can work for you if your goal is to build muscle and to get lean and here are 3 reasons why.

1. Recent studies have shown that it is in actual fact total macros and the total amount of daily calories that account for muscle growth and not the amount of meals and the timing of them. Essentially what this is saying is that as long as you get the required amount of calories in the 24 hour period it doesn't matter when you get them. So as long as you get you required amount of calories (a surplus of your TDEE is needed in combination with a progressive training routine) in your eating window you will gain muscle.

2. One facet of intermittent fasting bodybuilding that people complain about is the amount of food and calories that need to be consumed within the eaten window. Although you most likely will need to adjust if you are currently eating 6-8 small meals a day, over a period of a couple of weeks you stomach will adjust

to eating larger meals. I found it very difficult to eat large meals in the beginning but with in a week or so I adjusted and now I have no problems putting away large amounts of food in one sitting. Take your time with the adjustment period and don't expect to be able to switch over night.

3. Remember, like everything else intermittent fasting isn't an exact science and if you need to extend our eating window from say an eight hour eating window to a nine hour window to accommodate your total calories and meal requirements, that's fine go ahead and do so. Like any program it's important to find what works for you. Intermittent fasting, bodybuilding and building muscle can work together and the beauty of it is if you find that sweet spot that works for you you'll get the benefits of intermittent fasting while maintaining or building your physique to a bodybuilding level.

## Autophagy Restores Function in Aging Muscle Stem Cells

It has long been known that mesenchymal stem cells (MSCs) in skeletal muscle are an important part of the muscle repair process. Research has shown that exercise affects the behavior of your muscle stem cells, and may help prevent or even restore age-related muscle loss. MSCs in muscle are very responsive to mechanical strain, and these stem cells accumulate in muscle post-exercise.

And, while the MSCs do not directly contribute to building new muscle fibers, they do release growth factors, which encourage other cells to generate new muscle. It's also known that people's muscles tend to become increasingly deficient in MSCs with age, and that autophagy efficiency declines as well. As a result, metabolic waste starts to build up in your cells and tissues.

A recent study shows that satellite cells — muscle stem cells responsible for tissue regeneration — rely on autophagy to prevent the arrest of the cell cycle, known as cellular senescence; a state in which stem cell activity significantly declines. In short, to improve the regeneration of muscle tissue, you need to augment autophagy.

With efficient autophagy — your body's internal cleaning mechanism — your stem cells retain the ability to maintain and repair your tissues.

# CHAPTER SIX
## OPTIMIZING AUTOPHAGY

Autophagy can be affected by a number of factors that we control. When I discuss these measures with patients, it seems a bit overwhelming at first. But when we appreciate how far we've veered from our natural state of being, we recognize this is what it may take to truly optimize our bodies and brains.

### 1. Consider intermittent fasting.

Restriction of calories with intermittent fasting upregulates autophagy. Studies demonstrate caloric restriction is associated with an upregulation of autophagy in the liver, fat, brain, and muscle as well as being associated with longer, healthier life spans. This is thought to be due to increased availability of substrates and precursors for other essential biochemical reactions.

### 2. Eat more antioxidant-rich plants.

Intracellular enzymatic reactions require not only substrates but also co-factors for proper functioning. Co-factors are often vitamins that can be obtained from a wide array of plant-based foods. Excess protein and saturated fats, on the other hand, impair autophagy as they require too much cellular energy to

83

digest with a consequent increase in pro-inflammatory reactive oxygen species.

Plant-based foods contain a vast amount of antioxidants to reduce oxidative stress. Some key foods I recommend including in an overall plant-heavy diet are berries such as barberries, a source of the antioxidant berberine; broccoli seed sprouts, a source of sulforaphane; and green tea, a source of polyphenols. For a potent antioxidant fix, I also recommend juicing turmeric and ginger roots and drinking them daily. You should also avoid or scale way back on ultra-processed vegetable and seed oils (sunflower oil, palm oil, peanut oil, safflower oil, and soybean oil), saturated fat, sugar, and processed foods. These items are pro-inflammatory and can burden the mitochondria, impairing their function and role in autophagy.

### 3. Get that blood and oxygen flowing.

Regular aerobic exercise improves delivery of oxygen and nutrients to your cells by increasing blood flow to your vital organs. It also improves the transport of packaged and degraded inflammatory metabolites and waste by-products. Improving oxygenation has positive effects on autophagy and can also be accomplished by hyperbaric oxygen therapy (HBOT). HBOT helps wounds heal in part due to its regulation of autophagy. HBOT has also been shown to improve neurogenesis and decrease inflammation. An additional method of improving oxygenation and perfusion is compression technology equipment.

**4. Take steps to prioritize your sleep.**

The glymphatic system and autophagy are highly active during sleep. They work synergistically to improve the health and functioning of your brain. We should all work hard to respect the circadian nature of our brains and our bodies as this will help improve quality of sleep. It can be simple but requires motivation and dedication. Go to bed at the same time each night and wake at the same time each morning. Get outside in the morning for a dose of natural light. Eat at regular mealtimes and exercise at similar times each day. The use of melatonin 30 minutes prior to bedtime can also be helpful, and recent research supports this hormone's neuroprotective role.

**5. Amplify the AMPK pathway.**

The adenosine monophosphate-activated protein kinase (AMPK) is an enzyme that is critical for cellular bioenergetics. During nutrient-depleted states, AMPK is activated to upregulate autophagy so your body can maintain homeostatic demands. Impairment of the AMPK pathway has been associated with aging, cancer, neurodegenerative disease, and endocrine dysfunction.

So, how do you amplify it? Cold temperatures have been shown to upregulate AMPK, the basis behind cryotherapy, but could also be accomplished by cold showers, cold baths, cold swims, and the use of cold packs. There are also some natural medicines, such as cordyceps, that can regulate AMPK. Intermittent fasting and a diet low in saturated fats can be helpful as well.

## 6. Consider Exercise

Like the benefits of exercise, autophagy occurs in response to stress. And, in fact, exercise is one of the ways by which you boost autophagy. As you probably know, exercising creates mild damage to your muscles and tissues that your body then repairs, and by so doing makes your body stronger.

Exercise also helps flush out toxins by sweating, and is helpful for just about any detox program. In fact, many consider exercise a foundational aspect of effective detoxification.

Exercise is an important component as it also causes vasodilation and increased blood flow.

## HOW MUCH EXERCISE DO YOU NEED TO OPTIMIZE AUTOPHAGY?

The amount of exercise required to stimulate autophagy in humans is still unknown, however it is believed that intense exercise is more effective than mild exercise, which certainly makes logical sense.

That said, other research has shown that the "Goldilocks zone" in which exercise produces the greatest benefit for longevity is between 150 to 450 minutes of moderate exercise per week, lowering your risk of early death by 31 and 39 percent respectively. Spending at least 30 percent of your workout on high-intensity exercises has also been shown to further boost longevity by about 13 percent, compared to exercising at a consistently moderate pace all the time.

Following these general guidelines will likely put you in the most advantageous position for maximizing autophagy as well.

# CHAPTER SEVEN
## FULL BODY DETOX

It typically implies following a specific diet or using special products that claim to rid your body of toxins, thereby improving health and promoting weight loss.

Fortunately, your body is well-equipped to eliminate toxins and doesn't require special diets or expensive supplements to do so. That said, you can enhance your body's natural detoxification system.

**Misconceptions About Detoxing**

Detox diets are said to eliminate toxins from your body, improve health, and promote weight loss. They often involve the use of laxatives, diuretics, vitamins, minerals, teas, and other foods thought to have detoxing properties. The term "toxin" in the context of detox diets is loosely defined. It typically includes pollutants, synthetic chemicals, heavy metals, and processed foods — which all negatively affect health.

However, popular detox diets rarely identify the specific toxins they aim to remove or the mechanism by which they supposedly eliminate them. Moreover, no evidence supports the use of these diets for toxin elimination or sustainable weight loss. Your body has a sophisticated way of eliminating toxins that involves the liver, kidneys, digestive system, skin, and lungs. Still, only when these organs are healthy, can they effectively eliminate unwanted substances.

So, while detox diets don't do anything that your body can't naturally do on its own, you can optimize your body's natural detoxification system.

## 1. Limit Alcohol

More than 90% of alcohol is metabolized in your liver. Liver enzymes metabolize alcohol to acetaldehyde, a known cancer-causing chemical. Recognizing acetaldehyde as a toxin, your liver converts it to a harmless substance called acetate, which is later eliminated from your body.

While observational studies have shown low-to-moderate alcohol consumption beneficial for heart health, excessive drinking can cause a myriad of health problems. Excessive drinking can severely damage your liver function by causing fat buildup, inflammation, and scarring. When this happens, your liver cannot function adequately and perform its necessary tasks — including filtering waste and other toxins from your body.

As such, limiting or abstaining entirely from alcohol is one of the best ways to keep your body's detoxification system running strong. Health authorities recommend limiting alcohol intake to one drink per day for women and two for men. If you currently don't drink, you shouldn't start for the potential heart benefits associated with light-to-moderate drinking.

## 2. Focus on Sleep

Ensuring adequate and quality sleep each night is a must to support your body's health and natural detoxification system. Sleeping allows your brain to reorganize and recharge itself, as well as remove toxic waste byproducts that have accumulated throughout the day. One of those waste products is a protein called beta-amyloid, which contributes to the development of Alzheimer's disease . With sleep deprivation, your body does not have time to perform those functions, so toxins can build up and affect several aspects of health.

Poor sleep has been linked to short- and long-term health consequences, such as stress, anxiety, high blood pressure, heart disease, type 2 diabetes, and obesity. You should sleep seven to nine hours per night on a regular basis to promote good health. If you have difficulties staying or falling asleep at night, lifestyle changes like sticking to a sleep schedule and limiting blue light — emitted from mobile devices and computer screens — prior to bed are useful for improving sleep.

## 3. Drink More Water

Water does so much more than quench your thirst. It regulates your body temperature, lubricates joints, aids digestion and nutrient absorption, and detoxifies your body by removing waste products. Your body's cells must continuously be repaired to function optimally and break down nutrients for your body to use as energy.

However, these processes release wastes — in the form of urea and carbon dioxide — which cause harm if allowed to build up in your blood. Water transports these waste products, efficiently removing them through urination, breathing, or sweating. So staying properly hydrated is important for detoxification. The adequate daily intake for water is 125 ounces (3.7 liters) for men and 91 ounces (2.7 liters) for women. You may need more or less depending on your diet, where you live, and your activity level.

## 4. Reduce Your Intake of Sugar and Processed Foods

Sugar and processed foods are thought to be at the root of today's public health crises. High consumption of sugary and highly processed foods has been linked to obesity and other chronic diseases, such as heart disease, cancer, and diabetes. These diseases hinder your body's ability to naturally detoxify itself by harming organs that play an important role, such as your liver and kidneys. For example, high consumption of sugary beverages can cause fatty liver, a condition that negatively impacts liver function.

By consuming less junk food, you can keep your body's detoxification system healthy. You can limit junk food by leaving it on the store shelf. Not having it in your kitchen takes away the temptation altogether. Replacing junk food with healthier choices like fruits and vegetables is also a healthy way to reduce consumption.

## 5. Eat Antioxidant-Rich Foods

Antioxidants protect your cells against damage caused by molecules called free radicals. Oxidative stress is a condition caused by excessive production of free radicals. Your body naturally produces these molecules for cellular processes, such as digestion. However, alcohol, tobacco smoke, a poor diet, and exposure to pollutants can produce excessive free radicals.

By causing damage to your body's cells, these molecules have been implicated in a number of conditions, such as dementia, heart disease, liver disease, asthma, and certain types of cancer.

Eating a diet rich in antioxidants can help your body fight oxidative stress caused by excess free radicals and other toxins that increase your risk of disease.

Focus on getting antioxidants from food and not supplements, which may, in fact, increase your risk of certain diseases when taken in large amounts. Examples of antioxidants include vitamin A, vitamin C, vitamin E, selenium, lycopene, lutein, and zeaxanthin.

Berries, fruits, nuts, cocoa, vegetables, spices, and beverages like coffee and green tea have some of the highest amounts of antioxidants.

## 6. Eat Foods High in Prebiotics

Gut health is important for keeping your detoxification system healthy. Your intestinal cells have a detoxification and excretion system that protects your gut and body from harmful toxins, such as chemicals.

Good gut health starts with prebiotics, a type of fiber that feeds the good bacteria in your gut called probiotics. With prebiotics, your good bacteria are able to produce nutrients called short-chain fatty acids that are beneficial for health. The good bacteria in your gut can become unbalanced with bad bacteria from use of antibiotics, poor dental hygiene, and diet quality. Consequently, this unhealthy shift in bacteria can weaken your immune and detoxification systems and increase your risk of disease and inflammation. Eating foods rich in prebiotics can keep your immune and detoxification systems healthy. Good food sources of prebiotics include tomatoes, artichokes, bananas, asparagus, onions, garlic, and oats.

## 7. Decrease Your Salt Intake

For some people, detoxing is a means of eliminating excess water. Consuming too much salt can cause your body to retain excess fluid, especially if you have a condition that affects your kidneys or liver — or if you don't drink enough water. This excess fluid buildup can cause bloating and make clothing uncomfortable. If you find yourself consuming too much salt, you can detox yourself of the extra water weight. While it may sound counterintuitive, increasing your water intake is one of the best ways to eliminate excess water weight from consuming too much salt. That's because when you consume too much salt and not enough water, your body releases an antidiuretic hormone that prevents you from urinating — and therefore detoxifying.

By increasing your water intake, your body reduces the secretion of the antidiuretic hormone and increases urination, eliminating more water and waste products.

Increasing your intake of potassium-rich foods — which counterbalances some of sodium's effects — also helps. Foods rich in potassium include potatoes, squash, kidney beans, bananas, and spinach.

## 8. Get Active

Regular exercise, regardless of body weight is associated with a longer life and a reduced risk of many conditions and diseases, including type 2 diabetes, heart disease, high blood pressure, and certain cancers.

While there are several mechanisms behind the health benefits of exercise, reduced inflammation is a key point. While some inflammation is necessary for recovering from infection or healing wounds, too much of it weakens your body's systems and promotes disease.

By reducing inflammation, exercise can help your body's systems — including its detoxification system — function properly and protect against disease. It's recommended that you do at least 150–300 minutes a week of moderate-intensity exercise — such as brisk walking — or 75–150 minutes a week of vigorous-intensity physical activity — such as running.

## Other Helpful Detox Tips

Although no current evidence supports the use of detox diets for removing toxins from your body, certain dietary changes and lifestyle practices may help reduce toxin load and support your body's detoxification system.

- Eat sulfur-containing foods. Foods high in sulfur, such as onions, broccoli, and garlic, enhance excretion of heavy metals like cadmium.

- Try out chlorella. Chlorella is a type of algae that has many nutritional benefits and may enhance the elimination of toxins like heavy metals, according to animal studies.

- Flavor dishes with cilantro. Cilantro enhances excretion of certain toxins, such as heavy metals like lead, and chemicals, including phthalates and insecticides.

- Support glutathione. Eating sulfur-rich foods like eggs, broccoli, and garlic helps enhance the function of glutathione, a major antioxidant produced by your body that is heavily involved in detoxification.

- Switch to natural cleaning products. Choosing natural cleaning products like vinegar and baking soda over commercial cleaning agents can reduce your exposure to potentially toxic chemicals.

- Choose natural body care. Using natural deodorants, makeups, moisturizers, shampoos, and other personal care products can also reduce your exposure to chemicals.

While promising, many of these effects have only been shown in animal studies. Therefore, studies in humans are needed to confirm these findings.

## THE IMPORTANCE OF DETOXING BEFORE RESIDENTIAL TREATMENT

### Taking The First Step

One of the important steps that a person struggling with drug or alcohol addiction can take is to understand that they require help. It is this understanding that allows them to admit that can open doors to the best addiction treatment center for them and their health. It's important to understand what a rehab recovery program can actually do for a person struggling with addiction. One of the first steps that take place after an addict has signed up for an addiction recovery program is a drug detox.

Detoxification is the process in which all of the toxins that the drugs have introduced to the body are removed. It can be an extremely severe and unpleasant experience. That infamous experience is known as withdrawal, and all of its withdrawal symptoms can be especially difficult for an individual to get through on their own. However, it is a crucial step before other therapy methods can begin.

## Detox And Withdrawal

Once the individual has been admitted into the facility, they'll be supervised by a medical team or doctor 24/7. This is because withdrawal symptoms can be especially unpleasant and sometimes dangerous. While withdrawal varies from person to person and is dependent upon that person's health, the drugs typically used, and how long those drugs were used, overall, the symptoms can be difficult to deal with. In some cases, the withdrawal experience can even be deadly.

This is why a professional medical team is readily on hand to help the individual through every step of the drug detox process. In some cases, it may be prudent to offer them non-addictive pain medication or other types of medication that can assist them through the process. While the body is certainly going to be fighting its cravings, drug rehabs are not interested in hurting their patients—only helping and supporting them. Detox centers specialize in making the withdrawal symptoms as manageable as possible.

As such, it may be possible that a doctor offers the addict a form of medication to take the edge off of the more severe symptoms. Detoxing from alcohol and drugs typically associated with relieving symptoms of anxiety are perhaps some of the most difficult to detox from. They could lead to serious medical conditions such as cardiac arrest or seizures. Because of this, it's important that a person struggling with addiction seeks a detox from an actual addiction treatment center and not at home. Detoxing alone could prove lethal. Not to mention, detoxes performed at home are often less successful than those that are supervised by a knowledgeable and experienced team.

**After Detox**

Once the detox process has been completed, the toxins of the drugs or alcohol have completely left the body. It's likely that the addict will be feeling a little weak after the ordeal. However, they'll also likely feel a lot calmer and even healthier. Without detox, the body–and especially the brain–would be unable to move forward with the counseling that typically comes with the rest of the rehab recovery process.

Instead, if one did not go through a detox, it is likely that the brain, which has been hijacked by addiction, would cause the individual to seek out its addiction as soon as the therapy was over. In this case, time was spent receiving therapy, and they may have learned about triggers and environments that might lead them to use, but it wouldn't matter. Their brain is still addicted and craving the drug. This is because of drugs such as opium, heroin, and alcohol work on the pleasure receptors of the brain. The mind and body have become reliant on them, resulting in physical addiction.

This is different from the individual that received a detox. With their body free of the toxins, their mind is a bit clearer. While addiction is something that will likely always exist, it can be reduced. The brain can recover with time. However, it cannot recover if it is not free of toxic substances in the first place.

**Therapy**

Detox alone isn't enough to maintain a life of sobriety. Typically, those who only go through a detox and then jump right back into normal life have a higher risk of relapsing than those who stick through with the full program. This is because that while the body was able to remove its toxins, the behavior was not changed. So, when that particular individual was met with a situation where they were driven to take drugs or alcohol, they likely succumbed and relapsed.

The change in behavior comes from the numerous forms of therapy that rehab centers offer. There are group therapies as well as individual therapies. These two resources, in particular, can provide a safe place of support as well as understanding. For group therapies, individuals are able to meet with others who are going through the same situations and share their stories. Friendships can be made that can last even after the recovery program is over. In fact, it's suggested that these friendships remain strong after rehab so that the recovering individuals can continue to support one another in daily life.

For individual therapy, the recovering person can uncover the triggers and situations that drive them to take that drug or alcohol. If it's a toxic relationship, then they might seek counsel and support from their therapist to remove that toxicity from their lives. After all, personal physical and mental health is more important than a relationship that's unhealthy.

By uncovering these triggers, the individual can then develop healthy coping mechanisms, good behaviors, or even methods of avoidance to maintain their sobriety. With detox to rid their body of toxins, they can help their brain to heal. With therapy, they can learn good behaviors and understand their own triggers to better avoid relapsing. Together, these two halves of a recovery process can be extremely successful for an addicted individual. However, order matters. Without first detoxing, then an individual cannot hope to develop good behavior choices. They will only be a statistic of those who failed sobriety.

## THE IMPORTANCE OF MITOCHONDRIAL BIOGENESIS

Healthy mitochondria are at the core of staying healthy and preventing disease. Mitochondrial damage can trigger genetic mutations that can contribute to cancer, so optimizing the health of your mitochondria is a key component of cancer prevention. Autophagy is one way to remove damaged mitochondria, but biogenesis is the process by which new healthy mitochondria can be duplicated.

Interestingly, exercise plays a dual role as it not only stimulates autophagy but is also one of the most potent stimulators of mitochondrial biogenesis. It does this by increasing a signal in your body called AMPK, which in turn activates PGC-1 alpha.

By stimulating your mitochondria, the organelles in nearly every cell that produce ATP to work harder, your mitochondria start making reactive oxygen species (ROS), which act as signaling molecules. One of the functions they signal is to make more mitochondria.

In essence, the key to preventing disease virtually eliminating the risk of cancer, heart disease, diabetes, many other diseases and slowing down the aging process lies in optimizing mitochondrial function and increasing mitochondrial numbers. Thankfully, exercise helps you do both.

## KETOSIS DIET

keto diet is a popular diet containing high amounts of fats, adequate protein and low carbohydrate. It is also referred to as a Low Carb-High Fat (LCHF) diet and a low carbohydrate diet. It involves drastically reducing carbohydrate intake and replacing it with fat. This reduction in carbs puts the body into a metabolic state called ketosis.

When this happens, your body becomes incredibly efficient at burning fat for energy. It also turns fat into ketones in the liver, which can supply energy for the brain.

**What Is Ketosis?** - When the body is fueled completely by fat it enters a state called "Ketosis," which is a natural state for the body. After all of the sugars and unhealthy fats have been removed from the body during the first couple of weeks, the body is now free run on healthy fats.

Ketosis is the end result of a shift in the insulin/glucagon ratio and indicates an overall shift from a glucose based metabolism to a fat based metabolism. Ketosis occurs in a number of physiological states including fasting (called starvation ketosis), the consumption of a high fat diet (called dietary ketosis), and immediately after exercise (called post-exercise ketosis). Two pathological and potentially fatal metabolic states during which ketosis occurs are diabetic ketoacidosis and alcoholic ketoacidosis. The major difference between starvation, dietary and diabetic/alcoholic ketoacidosis is in the level of ketone concentrations seen in the blood. Starvation and dietary ketosis will normally not progress to dangerous levels, due to various feedback loops which are present in the body. Diabetic and alcoholic ketoacidosis are both potentially fatal conditions. All ketotic states ultimately occur for the same reasons. The first is a reduction of the hormone insulin and an increase in the hormone glucagon both of which are dependent on the depletion of liver glycogen. The second is an increase in FFA availability to the liver, either from dietary fat or the release of stored bodyfat.Under normal conditions, ketone bodies are present in the bloodstream in minute amounts, approximately 0.1 mmol/dl. When ketone body formation increases in the liver, ketones begin to accumulate in the bloodstream. Ketosis is defined clinically as a ketone concentration above 0.2 mmol/dl. Mild ketosis, around 2 mmol, also occurs following aerobic exercise.

## What Does Ketosis Represent?

The development of ketosis indicates two things. First, it indicates that the body has shifted from a metabolism relying primarily on carbohydrates for fuel to one using primarily fat and ketones for fuel.

This is arguably the main goal of the ketogenic diet: to cause an overall metabolic shift to occur in the body. Second, ketosis indicates that the entire pathway of fat breakdown is intact. The absence of ketosis under conditions which are known to induce it would indicate that a flaw in fat breakdown exists somewhere in the chain from fat breakdown, to transport, to oxidation in the liver. This absence would indicate a metabolic abnormality requiring further evaluation.

## What Causes Ketosis

When you start eating less amounts of carbohydrates, your body gets smaller supply of glucose to use as energy compared to before.

The decrease in the amount of consumed carbohydrates and the subsequent reduction in the amount of available glucose, slowly forces the body to move into the state of ketosis. Thus, the body goes into a state of ketosis when there is not enough amount of glucose available to the body cells.

## Starvation Induced Ketosis

Fasting and starvation states usually involve reduced or no intake of food that the body can digest and convert into glucose. While starvation is involuntary, fasting is a more conscious choice you make to intentionally not eat.

However, the body enters into a "starvation mode" whenever you are sleeping, when you skip a meal or when you intentionally go on a fast. The lack of food intake results in a reduction in blood glucose levels. As a result, the body starts to break down it glycogen (stored glucose) stores for energy.

The glycogen is converted back into glucose and used as energy by the body. In this state, the body also starts to burn its stored fats. Thus, the production of ketone bodies (ketogenesis) is induced by a lack of available glucose.

Any time the amount of ketones in the blood outnumber the molecules of glucose, the body cells will start making use of the ketones as their source of energy.

**Different Types of Ketogenic Diets**

There are several versions of the ketogenic diet, including:

• **Standard ketogenic diet (SKD):** This is a very low-carb, moderate-protein and high-fat diet. It typically contains 75% fat, 20% protein and only 5% carbs (1Trusted Source).

• **Cyclical ketogenic diet (CKD):** This diet involves periods of higher-carb refeeds, such as 5 ketogenic days followed by 2 high-carb days.

• **Targeted ketogenic diet (TKD):** This diet allows you to add carbs around workouts.

• **High-protein ketogenic diet:** This is similar to a standard ketogenic diet, but includes more protein. The ratio is often 60% fat, 35% protein and 5% carbs.

However, only the standard and high-protein ketogenic diets have been studied extensively. Cyclical or targeted ketogenic diets are more advanced methods and primarily used by bodybuilders or athletes.

There are several versions of the keto diet. The standard (SKD) version is the most researched and most recommended.

The information in this book mostly applies to the standard ketogenic diet (SKD), although many of the same principles also apply to the other versions.

## What Can You Eat on A Ketogenic Diet?

 A ketogenic diet is basically a diet which converts your body from burning sugar to burning fat. Around 99% of the wold's population have a diet which cause their body to burn sugar. As a result, carbohydrates are their primary fuel source used after digesting carbs. This process makes people gain weight, however a diet of fat and ketones will cause weight loss. As you ask what can you eat on a ketogenic diet, first of all eat up to 30 to 50 grams of carbs per day. Next, let us discover more about what you can have on your plate and how the ketogenic diet affects your health.

## The Importance of Sugar Precaution On The Ketogenic Diet

Keto shifts your body from a sugar burner to a fat burner by eliminating the dietary sugar derived from carbohydrates. The first obvious reduction you should make from your current diet is sugar and sugary foods. Although sugar is a definite target for deletion, the ketogenic diet focuses upon the limitation of carbohydrates. We need to watch out for sugar in a number of different types of foods and nutrients. Even a white potato which is carb-heavy may not taste sweet to your tongue like sugar. But once it hits your bloodstream after digestion, those carbs add the simple sugar known as glucose to your body. The truth is, our body can only store so much glucose before it dumps it elsewhere in our system. Excess glucose becomes what is known as the fat which accumulates in our stomach region, love handles, etc.

## Protein And It's Place In Keto

One source of carbohydrates which some people overlook in their diet is protein. Overconsumption of protein according to the tolerance level of your body will result in weight gain. Because our body converts excess protein into sugar, we must moderate the amount of protein we eat. Moderation of our protein intake is part of how to eat ketogenic and lose weight. First of all, identify your own tolerance of daily protein and use as a guide to maintain an optimal intake of the nutrient. Second, choose your protein from foods such as organic cage-free eggs and grass-fed meats. Finally, create meals in variety that are delicious and maintain your interest in the diet. For instance, a 5 ounce steak and a few eggs can provide an ideal amount of daily protein for some people.

## Caloric Intake on The Ketogenic Diet

Calories are another important consideration for what can you eat on a ketogenic diet. Energy derived from the calories in the food we consume help our body to remain functional. Hence, we must eat enough calories in order to meet our daily nutritional requirements. Counting calories is a burden for many people who are on other diets. But as a ketogenic dieter, you don't have to worry nearly as much about calorie counting. Most people on a low-carb diet remain satisfied by eating a daily amount of 1500-1700 kcals in calories.

## Fats, The Good & The Bad

Fat is not bad, in fact many good healthy fats exist in whole foods such as nuts, seeds and olive oil. Healthy fats are an integral part of the ketogenic diet and are available as spreads, snacks and toppings. Misconceptions in regards to eating fat are that a high amount of it is unhealthy and causes weight gain. While both statements are in a sense true, the fat which we consume is not the direct cause of the fat which appears on our body. Rather, the sugar from each nutrient we consume is what eventually becomes the fat on our body.

## Balance Your Nutrients Wisely

Digestion causes the sugars we eat to absorb into the bloodstream and the excess amount transfer into our fat cells. High carbohydrate and high protein eating will result in excess body fat, because there is sugar content in these nutrients. So excessive eating of any nutrient is unhealthy and causes weight gain. But a healthy diet consists of a balance of protein, carbohydrates and fats according to the tolerance levels of your body.

Just about everyone can accomplish a ketogenic diet with enough persistence and effort. In addition, we can moderate a number of bodily conditions naturally with keto. Insulin resistance, elevated blood sugar, inflammation, obesity, type-2 diabetes are some health conditions that keto can help to stabilize. Each of these unhealthy conditions will reduce and normalize for the victim who follows a healthy ketogenic diet. Low-carb, high-fat and moderate protein whole foods provide the life-changing health benefits of this diet.

## INSULIN AND KETOSIS

Insulin does a whole lot of different things, but it's best-known as the hormone that you make to metabolize carbs. Insulin gets a really bad rap in low-carb circles, to the point where it can get really oversimplified. There's more to weight gain than insulin! For general health, insulin isn't necessarily bad, and it's actually necessary for some health-related goals (for example, if you want to gain muscle, insulin is definitely your friend). But keto isn't just about general health. Keto is about a specific metabolic shift. If your goal is ketosis specifically, insulin is bad news – here's what you need to know.

### Insulin: Keto Enemy #1

The whole point of the ketogenic diet is that you're forcing your body to use ketone bodies for energy, instead of fat and carbohydrate. That's what makes the diet work.

Insulin suppresses ketone production. So if you want to get into ketosis and stay there, you want to minimize insulin as much as possible. Unless you're taking outside insulin, the easiest way to do this is by changing what you eat. Insulin is produced in response to different foods, so by changing your diet, you can minimize insulin production. That's the point of a ketogenic diet.

## Eating for Low Insulin Production

The ketogenic diet minimizes insulin production by restricting both carbs and protein – the diet keeps carbs as low as possible and supplies just enough protein to meet your needs, but not more.

### To reduce insulin production, lower carbs

Carbs raise insulin levels because you need insulin to metabolize carbs (use them for energy). The more carbs you eat, the more insulin you need.

**It works like this:** when you eat something carb-heavy, the glucose (carbohydrate) in that food raises your blood sugar. But having high blood sugar all the time is dangerous, so when your body senses that you've eaten carbohydrates, your pancreas makes some insulin to take that glucose out of the bloodstream and store it somewhere safe (your fat cells) for later use.

This is all fine and good, and if you're going to eat carbs, you want it to work exactly like that. If you eat carbs but can't produce enough insulin (e.g. people with type 1 diabetes), you'll be in very deep trouble. But the flip side of this is that if you want to reduce insulin production, you've got to lower carbs.

## To reduce insulin production, lower protein

This one is a bit more of a surprise – most people know that carbs have something to do with Protein powderinsulin, but not a lot of people know that protein can also trigger an insulin spike. But it's true!

For example, in this study, adding whey protein to a mixed meal increased the insulin response to the meal. Other types of dairy protein are also insulinogenic – that's why keto focuses on high-fat, low-protein dairy foods (like butter), not high-protein, low-fat dairy foods (like Greek yogurt). It's all about reducing the insulin spike.

It's not totally clear how protein causes this insulin response. It's possible that protein causes an insulin spike by stimulating the secretion of another protein, GLP-1, which then goes on to stimulate insulin secretion.

What is clear is that if you want a diet that minimizes insulin production, you'd also want to reduce protein. In practice, it's not practical or even desirable to get protein down to almost nothing, the way you can with carbs. Protein does more than just cause insulin spikes, and protein deficiency causes problems of its own. So on keto, the goal is to have adequate protein: enough to keep you healthy and meet all your needs, but not more.

## Keto: low in carbs, moderate in protein

All of this research on carbs, protein, and insulin explains the whys and hows of keto pretty well. If the goal is to use ketones for energy, you need to reduce insulin production, which means minimizing carbs, reducing protein by quite a bit, and relying mostly on fat for calories because, well, fat is what you have left. Fat raises insulin levels very minimally, especially if it's not in the context of overeating. A high-fat, adequate-protein, low-carb diet doesn't totally prevent insulin production, but it reduces it by enough that the very low level of insulin left doesn't stop you from making ketone bodies.

And the results are pretty impressive. Eating a keto diet significantly reduces fasting insulin and postprandial insulin (insulin levels right after a meal). In patients with diabetes who rely on outside insulin, a ketogenic diet reduces the need for insulin.

## Keto, Insulin Resistance, and Insulin Sensitivity

On the topic of keto and insulin in general, it's worth noting how keto affects insulin sensitivity and insulin resistance.

Insulin gets glucose out of your bloodstream (where it's dangerous) and into your muscles, liver, and fat tissue (where it's not). But for insulin to do that effectively, it has to be able to "persuade" all of these tissues to let the glucose in.

In people who are insulin sensitive, these other tissues are receptive to the insulin signal: they're happy to open the door when insulin comes knocking. In people who are insulin resistant, these tissues resist the insulin signal. If insulin can't do its job, all that glucose stays right in the bloodstream (after all, where else is it going to go?) and the insulin resistant person ends up with high blood sugar all the time. When this gets diagnosed as an actual disease, it's called type 2 diabetes.

Now take a look at what happens when you throw a keto diet into that mix. Blood sugar control improves and people can reduce the amount of insulin they have to take as medication. This is especially true for people with higher blood sugar to begin with. Keto is impressively therapeutic for people with insulin resistance and problems controlling their blood sugar – on top of people with type 2 diabetes, it also works for women with polycystic ovary syndrome (PCOS), another disease that's marked by insulin resistance.

Basically, because a keto diet doesn't require you to be able to make insulin or use it normally, it's very therapeutic for people who can't do that.

## How Long Does It Take To Get Into Ketosis And Keto Adapt?

Keto-adaptation (also sometimes called fat-adaptation) is the process your body goes through on the diet as it changes from using primarily glucose for energy to using primarily fat.

The "keto" part refers to ketones, which are water-soluble molecules that the liver makes when metabolizing fats, particularly when carbohydrate intake is low. Ketones can be used for energy by most tissues in your body, including the brain, which can't use unrefined fats as fuel.

Your body is always using a mix of fat and glucose for energy, but in a non-keto-adapted state, it reaches for glucose first, since only low amounts of ketones are normally generated during fat metabolism and some tissues of the body—for example, the heart—prefer using ketones when they're available. The brain can't use fat, so it depends on glucose when you're in a non-keto-adapted state.

If glucose is the body's normal go-to source of energy, you may be wondering what happens when it suddenly doesn't have enough to use as its main fuel.

## Getting to a Keto-Adaptive State

Once stores of glycogen (the way the body warehouses glucose) become depleted, your brain and other organs begin the process of adapting to using fats and ketones instead of glucose as its main fuel. But reaching ketosis, the state in which fat provides most of the fuel for your body, isn't usually a pleasant experience.

The extreme carb restriction is often accompanied by adverse side effects. Commonly known as the "keto flu," the transition may cause a period of fatigue, weakness, lightheadedness, "brain fog," headaches, irritability, muscle cramps, and nausea.

While the length of time it takes to adapt to a keto diet varies, the process begins after the first few days. Then, after about a week to 10 days, many low-carbers suddenly start to feel the positive effects of keto-adaptation. They report improved mental concentration and focus and more physical energy as well.

By the end of the second week (sometimes up to three weeks), the body has usually accomplished the majority of its work in adapting to using fat for energy. By this point, hunger and food cravings are diminished and stamina and vitality increased.

After this, the body continues to make more subtle changes. For example, it gradually becomes more conserving of protein, so people often crave less protein. Another change that athletes often notice is less lactic acid buildup in their muscles with long training sessions, which translates into less fatigue and soreness. It can take up to 12 weeks for these changes to occur and for you to fully reach ketosis.

**Helping Your Body Adapt**

There are a number of ways you can get over the hurdle of the first week of carbohydrate withdrawal:

- **Eat lots of fat and fiber.** The fuller you feel, the less likely you are to miss your favorite carb-laden foods. Foods made with flaxseeds are high in both fiber and healthy omega-3 fats.

- **Increase salt and water intake.** Many of the negative side effects are caused by a loss of fluid and electrolytes like sodium (carbs hold on to water, so you'll probably urinate a lot more once you cut them out). To replenish both, drink a cup of water with a half teaspoon of salt stirred into it or a cup of bouillon several times a day for a few days.

- **Go easy with physical activity.** As you adapt to a new fuel source, strenuous workouts can further stress your body, so stick to gentle forms of exercise like walking and stretching for a few weeks.

## How Long Does It Take to Reach Fat Adaptation?

It generally takes from 30 days to 12 weeks of sticking to a keto diet to become fat adapted. During this time you want to focus on clean whole foods and sticking to eating a ketogenic diet without cheats or deviations.

First, you'll experience the initial phase: carb withdrawal, which lasts anywhere from 3 to 14 days and is characterized by cravings, hunger, and perhaps the keto flu. Then you'll roll right into the second phase, where your body is adjusting from relying on glucose for energy to relying on fat, which can last 6 to 8 weeks. After several weeks, your body is on fat-burning autopilot, and that's where you'll stay as long as you maintain a keto lifestyle!

### Signs That You're Fat Adapted

How will you know when you've made the final transformation from traditional sugar burner to fat burner? When you:

- Can go 4 to 6 hours between meals without getting hungry

- Feel consistently energetic throughout the day, without energy slumps or a rumbling tummy

- Can easily work out while remaining on a keto diet

**Managing Keto-Adaptation**

Some people find that their ketosis is pretty stable as long as they eat a low-carb diet under about 50 grams of carbs a day, while others find they need to eat fewer carbs to stay in ketosis. Athletes and heavy exercisers often can eat more than 50 grams of carbs and still stay in ketosis. Other influences, such as hormonal fluctuations and stress, have been known to throw people out of ketosis.

Some people find value in measuring their blood ketones, which can be done at home using a special meter and test strips.

If you're getting the benefits you hoped for on a keto diet, worrying about how high your ketones are, may just add a level of complication you don't need.

# CHAPTER EIGHT
## AUTOPHAGY: A CURE FOR MANY PRESENT-DAY DISEASES

Autophagy, a cellular cleaning process, gets activated in response to certain types of metabolic stress, including nutrient deprivation, growth factor depletion and hypoxia. Even without adequate circulation, each cell may break down sub-cellular parts and recycle those into new proteins or energy as required to survive. This explains why mTOR and autophagy are seen in every organism from yeast to humans.

Studies on mutations of animals as varied as yeast, slime molds, plants and mice show that deletions of autophagy-related genes (ATG) in animals is largely incompatible with life. That is, most life on earth cannot survive without autophagy.

Insulin and amino acids (through mTOR) are the main regulators of ATGs. These also happen to be two of our most basic nutrient sensors. When we eat carbohydrates, insulin goes up. When we eat protein, both insulin and mTOR go up. When nutrient sensors sense, well, nutrients, we signal our body to grow bigger, not to get smaller. Thus nutrient sensors turn off autophagy, which is primarily a catabolic (breaking down) as opposed to an anabolic (building up) process. However, there is a low basal level of autophagy going on at all times, as it acts as a sort of a cellular housekeeper.

**Cellular housekeeper**

Autophagy's main roles are:

- Remove defective proteins and organelles
- Prevent abnormal protein aggregate accumulation
- Remove intracellular pathogens

These mechanisms are implicated in many aging-related diseases – atherosclerosis, cancer, Alzheimer's disease, neurodegenerative diseases (Parkinsons). There is a basal cellular housekeeping provides quality control on the proteins in our body. Mice genetically mutated lacking ATGs develop excess protein buildup inside cells. There is both too much protein, and damaged proteins that are not broken down. It's sort of like the junk you have in the basement. If you have some old, broken down lawn furniture, you should probably toss it into the dumpster. If you keep it around in your basement, soon your house starts to look like that TV show 'Hoarders'. There is a related process called mitophagy to cull the abnormal organelles (mitochondria, in this case).

**Autophagy: a tumor suppressor?**

In cancer, it is generally accepted that autophagy can suppress tumor initiation. Since autophagy blocks growth and increases breakdown of proteins, this makes perfect sense. Cancer cells, for example, often have much lower levels of basal autophagy than normal cells. Many of the best-studied oncogenes and tumor-suppressor genes are intimately associated with autophagy.

For example, the well known PTEN tumor-suppressor gene blocks PI3K/Akt thus activating autophagy. Mutations to PTEN, found very commonly in cancers, thus lead to lower levels of autophagy and increased risk of cancer. However, it appears to be a double-edged sword. As cancer progresses, autophagy may help cancer survival, just as it helps all cells survive in a stressful environment.

During times of low nutrients, autophagy breaks down proteins for amino acids, which may be used for energy. Cancer, which may grow so quickly as to outstrip its own blood supply, may thus be aided by increased autophagy, as this would supply much needed energy and deal with stress.

**Neurodegenerative diseases**

The other area of intense interest is the neurodegenerative diseases of Alzheimer's Disease,

Parkinson's disease and Huntington's chorea. While these all manifest differently, Alzheimer's with loss of memory and other cognitive changes, Parkinson's with loss of voluntary movement and resting tremor and Huntington's with involuntary movements, they all share one pathologic similarity.

All these diseases are characterized by excessive build up of proteins inside neurons leading to dysfunction and ultimately disease. Thus, failure of protein degradation pathways may play a very important role in preventing these diseases. However, the exact role of autophagy in these diseases is still yet to be defined. Further, growing research also implicates mitochondrial dysfunction as a key pathway in the development of neurodegenerative diseases.

Studies in humans are difficult to do because of the multiple intersecting pathways. The clearest evidence usually comes from drugs where a single pathway can be changed at a time. The mTOR inhibitors (rapamycin, everolimus) activate autophagy by blocking mTOR. Remember that mTOR is a nutrient sensor, predominantly for amino acids. If there is protein being eaten, mTOR goes up, and growth pathways are allowed to continue. If there are no nutrients being eaten, mTOR goes down, and autophagy goes up. Rapamycin blocks mTOR, fooling the body into thinking that there are no nutrients and this increases autophagy.

These drugs are mainly used for the their immune-suppressing effects in transplant medicine. Interestingly, though, most immune suppressants increase the risk of cancer where rapamycin does not. In certain rare cancers, mTOR inhibitors have demonstrated anti-cancer effects.

Metformin, a drug widely used in type 2 diabetes, also activates autophagy but not through mTOR. It increases AMPK, a molecule that signals the energy status of the cell. If AMPK is high, the cell knows that it has insufficient energy and increases autophagy. AMPK senses the ADP/ATP ratio, thus knowing the cellular energy levels – sort of like a fuel gauge but in reverse. High AMPK, low cellular energy status. High AMPK levels directly and indirectly activate autophagy, but also mitochondrial production.

## Mitophagy

Mitophagy is the selective targeting of defective or dysfunctional mitochondrion. These are the parts of the cell that produce energy – the power houses. If these are not working properly, then the process of mitophagy targets them for destruction. The critical regulators of this process includes the notorious tumor suppressor gene PTEN. This may initially seem bad, remember that, at the same time that mitophagy is increased, new mitochondrion are being stimulated to grow. AMPK for example, will stimulate mitophagy as well as new mitochondrion growth – essentially replacing old mitochondrion with new ones in a renewal process. This is fantastic – essentially a complete renovation of the mitochondrial pool. Break down the old, junky mitochondrion and stimulate the body to build new ones. This is one of the reasons metformin is commonly promoted as an anti-aging compound – not so much for its blood-sugar effects, but instead because of its effect on AMPK and autophagy.

Notice how mTOR is the most central nutrient sensor to impact autophagy. mTOR integrates signals from insulin, nutrients (amino acids or dietary protein) and the fuel gauge of the cell, AMPK (all energy including fats) to determine whether the cell should divide and grow, or involute and become dormant. Excess nutrients – not merely carbohydrates, but all nutrients may stimulate the mTOR system and thus turn off autophagy, putting the body into a growth mode. This encourages growth of cells, which, as I will repeat often, is not usually good in adults.

These pathways are central to life on earth because they are the link between nutrient status and growth. For single-celled organisms, if there was not enough nutrients, they simply went into a dormant stage. Think about a yeast. If there is no food, it simply dries up into a spore. When it lands on water, it blooms and starts to grow. So mold is sitting in your house in a dried up, inactive state. If it lands on some bread, it starts to grow into a familiar mold. It only grows when there are sufficient nutrients and water.

In a multi-celled organism, it becomes much more difficult to synchronize the availability of nutrients and growth signalling. Consider an animal such as a human being. We are designed to live for days or weeks without food – subsisting on the stored food energy in our body fat. However, when food is scarce, we do not want to grow quickly and therefore we require nutrient sensors which are directly connected to growth pathways. The main three are:

- mTOR – sensitive to dietary protein

- AMPK – 'reverse fuel gauge' of the cell

- Insulin – sensitive to protein and carbohydrates

When these nutrient sensors detect low nutrient availability, they tell our cells to stop growing and start breaking down unnecessary parts – this is the self cleansing pathway of autophagy. Here's the critical part. If we have diseases of excessive growth, then we can reduce growth signalling by activating these nutrient sensors. This list of diseases includes – obesity, type 2 diabetes, Alzheimer's disease, cancer, atherosclerosis (heart attacks and strokes), polycystic ovarian syndrome, polycystic kidney disease and fatty liver disease, among others. All these diseases are amenable to dietary intervention, not more drugs.

## THE IMPACTS OF AUTOPHAGY ON HUMAN PHYSIOLOGY AND DISEASES

Nearly all eukaryotic cells undergo autophagy at a basal level under normal physiological conditions, and cells deficient in autophagy show diffuse abnormal protein accumulation and mitochondria disorganization, suggesting that cells use autophagy to maintain cellular homeostasis by eliminating damaged organelles and protein aggregates, which resist degradation via UPS in normal growing conditions. In addition to the effect on cellular homeostasis maintenance, autophagy also regulates rapid cellular changes essential for mammalian development and differentiation. For instance, it has been demonstrated that autophagy is required in mitochondrial elimination during erythrocyte and adipocyte maturation. Furthermore, autophagy is not only responsible for the clearance of abnormal proteins and organelles, but also participates in the removing of infectious agents, including bacteria and viruses from host cells. Recent data from studies of cell models show that autophagy upregulation might be valuable for eliminating Mycobacterium tuberculosis , Streptococcus, mycobacteria and herpes simplex virus.

This function of autophagy appears to be accounted for by both innate and adaptive immune responses.

Because of the importance of autophagy in mammalian physiology, it is therefore reasonable to assume that autophagy impairment could contribute to human diseases. However, although autophagy was first described morphologically in mammalian cells in 1960s, until the discovery of a group of autophagy-related (ATG) genes in 1990s, the role of autophagy in various human disease states was unclear, and only in the past decade has the connection between autophagy and human disease become the subject of intense study. To date, autophagy has been linked to a growing list of diseases, and it appears that more autophagy-associated diseases will be discovered in the future. Although the exact mechanisms underlying the autophagy-associated diseases at the molecular level remain not fully understood, the recent advances in autophagy research present a potential target for manipulation of autophagy in human diseases. The following reviews aim at outlining our current understanding of mechanisms involved in autophagy activation, and its important roles in human physiology and diseases, including diabetes mellitus, neurodegenerative disorders, infectious diseases and cancer

## Autophagy in disease

The broad array of physiological functions attributed to autophagy justifies why alterations in this catabolic process lead to cellular malfunctioning and often cell death. Autophagy has been widely implicated in many pathophysiological processes such as cancer, metabolic and neurodegenerative disorders as well as cardiovascular and pulmonary diseases. It also has an important role in aging and exercise.

## Neurodegenerative diseases

Neurodegenerative diseases are characterized by accumulation of mutant or toxic proteins. It has been shown that autophagic pathway helps in cell survival by removing unwanted cellular organelle and protein aggregates. Disruption of autophagy specific genes in neural cells lead to neurodegeneration.

## Autophagic dysfunction in neurodegenerative disorders

As AD progresses, either due to AD related genes or environmental/aging factors, several pathological changes of the lysosomal network occurs, such as deregulation of endocytosis and increased lysosomal biogenesis culminating in a progressive failure of lysosomal clearance mechanisms. Enlargement of Rab5 and Rab7 positive endosomes is one of the earliest specific pathology reported in AD brain tissue which reflects a pathological acceleration of endocytosis. Interestingly, it develops in pyramidal neurons of the neocortex at a stage when plaques and tangles are restricted only to the hippocampus. Furthermore genes involved in endocytosis are up-regulated in AD and their corresponding proteins are abnormally recruited to endosomes promoting fusion and enlargement of early and late endosomes, which is a specific characteristic of AD and is not seen in normal aging brain. Acceleration of endosome pathology is also seen in individuals who inherit the ε4 allele of APOE, the major risk factor

for late-onset AD. Lipinski and co-workers recently reported that transcription of factors that promote autophagy are up-regulated in the brains of AD patients, while negative regulators of autophagy are down-regulated. Indeed, cellular ultrastructural changes have been described in AD brain biopsies revealing a high level of AVs within dystrophic neurites. AVs and lysosomes constitute more than 95% of the organelles in dystrophic neuritic swellings in AD. This means that autophagy initiation is up-regulated or its progression is either delayed or impaired. However the profuse and selective accumulation of AVs in dystrophic neurites indicates a defect in the clearance of AVs by lysosomes rather than an abnormally augment of autophagy. In the case of familial AD, for instance, presenilin 1 (a ubiquitous transmembrane protein involved in diverse biological roles) mutations hinder lysosome proteolysis and accelerate neuritic dystrophy which also supports a primary role for failure of proteolytic clearance. Presenilin 1 is required for lysosome acidification which is needed to activate cathepsins and other hydrolases that carry out digestion during autophagy.

Mutations in Presenilin 1 result in impaired targeting of the a1 subunit of V0-ATPase from the endoplasmic reticulum to the lysosome. As V0-ATPase is required for acidification of the autolysosome contents, mutations in Presenilin 1 are proposed to be involved in the defective proteolysis of autophagic substrates in patients with AD. Furthermore, Zhang and colleagues reported for the first time, a role for presenilins in regulating lysosomal biogenesis. The role of impaired lysosomal degradation in the etiology of AD was underscored in a study of a transgenic mouse model of this disease. In these mice, deletion of cystatin B (an endogenous inhibitor of lysosomal cysteine proteases) stimulated the turnover of proteins by the lysosome, enhanced the clearance of the autophagic substrates, and rescued the deficient cognitive phenotype of the animals. Furthermore, in APP transgenic mouse models of AD, undigested autophagic substrates. This general failure to clear autophagy substrates affects clearance of various proteins relevant to AD pathogenesis, including the protein Aβ 92 Autophagy - A Double-Edged Sword - Cell Survival or Death? and tau promoting cell death. These results indicate that mutant APP overexpression alone can lead to autophagic-lysosomal pathology. However the mechanism by which overexpres- sion of mutant APP may lead to impaired autophagy and neuritic dystrophy, is not well understood. One possibility is that APP may affect the endosomal-lysosomal system. Strong overexpression of human Aβ42 in Drosophila neurons induces age-related accumulation of Aβ in AVs and neurotoxicity which is further enhanced by autophagy activation and is partially rescued by autophagy inhibition. These authors propose that the structural integrity of post-fusion AVs may be compromised in Aβ42 affected neurons, leading to subcellular damage and loss of neuronal integrity in the Aβ42 flies. Moreover, expression of an APOEε4 allele, but not the APOEε3 allele, in a mouse AD model increases levels of intracellular Aβ in lysosomes, altering their function and causing neurodegeneration. Interestingly, inhibition of Aβ aggregation rescues the autophagic deficits in the TgCRND8 mouse model of AD. Autophagy sequesters and digests unneeded or damaged organelles, some of which are APP-rich. Autophagosomes are enriched in APP as well as APP substrates and enzymes that are responsible for processing APP into Aβ. Under normal circunstances Aβ is subsequently degraded by lysosomes. Therefore autophagosomes are a site of intracellular production of Aβ, thus upon their cellular accumulation amyloid deposition occurs. Failure of the autophagic system also compromises the elimination of aggregate forms of tau, a protein that also accumulates in AD neurons. In fact, for certain types of tau mutations, pathogenic tau could contribute to the failure of macroautophagy, due to the toxic effect that the still soluble forms of the protein exert in the membrane of lysosomes when they are delivered to this compartment by CMA. Furthermore, particular mutant forms of tau have been shown to abnormally interact with components of the lysosomal CMA translocation machinery. More interestingly, stimulation of autophagy is neuroprotective in a mouse model of human tauopathy. In addition to the defects in late stages of autophagy, evidence suggests that autophagy might be disrupted at the level of autophagosome formation in patients with AD. Compared with healthy individuals, the brains of patients with AD show reduced expression of Beclin-1, which could lead to an impairment in the initiation of autophagy. Transgenic mice that expressed a mutated form of the human APP on a Beclin-1 haploinsufficient background had disrupted autophagy, as well as, increased intracellular Aβ accumulation and neurodegeneration, compared with mice that expressed the mutated human APP in the context of a normal Beclin-1 background. Caspase 3-mediated cleavage of Beclin-1 occurs in the brains of patients with AD; thus, increased activity of this enzyme might contribute to the loss of Beclin-1 function in individuals with this disease.

## Cancer

Autophagy was first linked to cancer through the role of Beclin , which is essential for autophagy pathway, and has been mapped to tumor susceptibility. Since then, a number of tumor-suppressor proteins have been identified that are involved in control of autophagy pathway

The tumor cells exploit the autophagic mechanism to provide a way for them to overcome nutrient-limiting conditions and facilitate tumor growth. Studies show that autophagy can modulate the tumor microenvironment by promoting angiogenesis, supply nutrients, and modulate inflammatory response

## Cardiovascular diseases

Autophagic pathway is essential for normal maintenance, repair, and adaptation of the heart tissue. Unsurprisingly therefore, autophagic deficiencies have been associated with a variety of cardiac pathologies.

Infectious disease Autophagy plays a key role in immune defence against invading bacteria and pathogens. Upon infection, autophagy regulates inflammation, antigen presentation and micro-organism capture and degradation.

# CHAPTER NINE
## COMMON MYTHS AND QUESTIONS
## OF INTERMITTENT FASTING

Because there are different types of intermittent fasting and no specific authority or dedicated source for information, there are quite a few myths about the eating style.

**Myth 1** - You Must Eat 3 Meals Per Day: This "rule" that is common in Western society was not developed based on evidence for improved health, but was adopted as the common pattern for settlers and eventually became the norm. Not only is there a lack of scientific rationale in the 3 meal-a-day model, recent studies may be showing less meals and more fasting to be optimal for human health. One study showed that one meal a day with the same amount of daily calories is better for weight loss and body composition than 3 meals per day. This finding is a basic concept that is extrapolated into intermittent fasting and those choosing to do IF may find it best to only eat 1-2 meals per day.

**Myth 2** - You Need Breakfast, It's The Most Important Meal of The Day: Many false claims about the absolute need for a daily breakfast have been made. The most common claims being "breakfast increases your metabolism" and "breakfast decreases food intake later in the day". These claims have been refuted and studied over a 16 week period with results showing that skipping breakfast did not decrease metabolism and it did not increase food intake at lunch and dinner. It is still possible to do intermittent fasting protocols while still eating breakfast, but some people find it easier to eat a late breakfast or skip it altogether and this common myth should not get in the way.

## Myth 3 - Intermittent fasting is more effective for weight loss than traditional diets.

Current evidence suggests that those who follow traditional calorie-restriction diets lose about the same amount of weight as those who follow intermittent fasting programs. Several studies have found that while there is a slight advantage for those doing IF, the advantage isn't significant. Additionally, experts still don't know if IF programs are sustainable.

## Myth 4 - Intermittent fasting causes muscle loss.

Starvation can cause a loss of lean muscle tissue. So, it would seem reasonable to assume that intermittent fasting would also cause some degree of muscle wasting. However, the evidence so far has shown that intermittent fasting may spare muscle when compared to conventional dieting.

In a 2011 review, 90 percent of the weight lost through intermittent fasting was fat (rather than muscle), compared with only 75 percent in daily dieting. This would suggest that conventional dieting causes greater muscle loss than IF programs.

Maintaining lean muscle mass while dieting offers a metabolic advantage for trying to maintain weight loss because muscle burns more energy than fat even at rest.

## Myth 5- Intermittent fasting works better for losing belly fat

Belly fat, also known as visceral fat, is the spare tire that surrounds your internal organs, leading to a greater risk of diabetes and heart disease. A 2011 review found that both traditional dieting and intermittent fasting reduce similar amounts of belly fat.

## Myth 6 - Intermittent fasting will improve your level of fitness.

Some people believe that the human body maximizes fat loss and cardio efficiency in a fasted state during aerobic exercise first thing in the morning. The practice—called fasted cardio—has caught on in certain fitness communities. However, there isn't a lot of scientific evidence to support the practice

## Myth 7- You'll live longer if you practice intermittent fasting.

This is one of the most widely held beliefs by many people who adhere to an intermittent fasting protocol. But there hasn't been enough research conducted on humans to know if it is a fact, according to the National Institutes of Health Institute on Aging.

Rodent studies have suggested that intermittent fasting boosts longevity. But humans have very different lifestyles than mice and those differences have substantial implications. The bottom line is that we don't know how intermittent fasting affects human longevity.

## COMMON QUESTIONS ABOUT INTERMITTENT FASTING:

Here are answers to the most common questions about intermittent fasting.

## 1. Can I Drink Liquids During the Fast?

Yes. Water, coffee, tea and other non-caloric beverages are fine. Do not add sugar to your coffee. Small amounts of milk or cream may be okay.

Coffee can be particularly beneficial during a fast, as it can blunt hunger.

## 2. Isn't It Unhealthy to Skip Breakfast?

No. The problem is that most stereotypical breakfast skippers have unhealthy lifestyles. If you make sure to eat healthy food for the rest of the day then the practice is perfectly healthy.

## 3. Can I Take Supplements While Fasting?

Yes. However, keep in mind that some supplements like fat-soluble vitamins may work better when taken with meals.

## 4. Can I Work out While Fasted?

Yes, fasted workouts are fine. Some people recommend taking branched-chain amino acids (BCAAs) before a fasted workout.

## 5. Will Fasting Cause Muscle Loss?

All weight loss methods can cause muscle loss, which is why it's important to lift weights and keep your protein intake high. Studies show that intermittent fasting causes less muscle loss than regular calorie restriction

## 6. Will Fasting Slow Down My Metabolism?

No. Studies show that short-term fasts actually boost metabolism . However, longer fasts of 3 or more days can suppress metabolism.

## 7. Should Kids Fast?

Allowing your child to fast is probably a bad idea.

## TESTIMONIAL

Intermittent Fasting and what it has done for me!

I have performed this for the last 9 months, and it has worked wonders for me, and is a great new lifestyle that I am following, and will not ever change from this, as it has way too many great benefits! This is not something you start and do, and then stop once you are happy, it is a way of life, which is easily maintainable, and helps you to eat anything you like as well! If you can maintain this consistently over your life, you will always stay lean and healthy, something which I have achieved from this and will continue to do so. This method piled on with exercise as well will only guarantee great results in the long term and short term. Only try this method if you know you can! If you find the fact of fasting and staying away from food too hard, then please do look at something else you will feel comfortable with, but this is my view, and is a great method if you do choose to follow it.

**This Is Crazy. If I Didn't Eat For 24 Hours, I'd Die.**

Honestly, I think the mental barrier is the biggest thing that prevents people from fasting because it's really not that hard to do in practice.

Here are a few reasons why intermittent fasting isn't as crazy as you think it is.

First, fasting has been practiced by various religious groups for centuries. Medical practitioners have also noted the health benefits of fasting for thousands of years. In other words, fasting isn't some new fad or crazy marketing ploy. It's been around for a long time and it actually works. Second, fasting seems foreign to many of us simply because nobody talks about it that much. The reason for this is that nobody stands to make much money by telling you to not eat their products, not take their supplements, or not buy their goods. In other words, fasting isn't a very marketable topic and so you're not exposed to advertising and marketing on it very often. The result is that it seems somewhat extreme or strange, even though its really not.

Third, you've probably already fasted many times, even though you don't know it. Have you ever slept in late on the weekends and then had a late brunch? Some people do this every weekend. In situations like these, we often eat dinner the night before and then

143

don't eat until 11am or noon or even later. There's your 16–hour fast and you didn't even think about it.

Finally, I would suggest doing one 24–hour fast even if you don't plan on doing intermittent fasting frequently. It's good to teach yourself that you'll survive just fine without food for a day.

# **CONCLUSION**

Autophagy is nature's way of allowing your body to cleanse and heal itself, and that rest is paramount to the success of the process. Our health depends on our healthy cells, that is why our body uses autophagy to revitalize our cells. Autophagy is a cell renewal process that works as your body's housekeeper. Autophagy may be able to delay the effects of aging, protect against mutation and loss of function, and help in preventing diseases such as Parkinson's, Alzheimer's, cancer, and heart disease.

Autophagy is induced mainly through a reduction in insulin and an increase in glucagon where glucagon then acts to induce autophagy. Other mechanisms, such as a reduction in TOR kinase, which blocks autophagy, also works to increase autophagy in the body. Diet and exercise routines offer the easiest route to increasing autophagy, with intermittent fasting, ketosis, and increased exercise all increasing glucagon and autophagy levels.

The amount of time we live is called lifespan. The length of time that a person is healthy and functional not just alive is called healthspan.

Intermittent fasting is valuable for effecting both lifespan (in studied organisms but not yet proven in humans) and the healthspan (in organisms including humans).

It is common within the aging and longevity space to focus on lifespan to the detriment of quality of life.

In contrast, the length of time that a person is healthy and functional is correlated with higher quality of life. Healthspan can be mediated by dietary interventions and exercise

## Health and Longevity Are Rooted in Mitochondrial Function

The take-home message here is that your lifestyle determines your fate in terms of how long you'll live and, ultimately, how healthy those years will be. For optimal health and disease prevention, you need healthy mitochondria and efficient autophagy (cellular cleaning and recycling), and three key lifestyle factors that have a beneficial effect on both are:

**What you eat:** A diet high in quality fats, moderate in protein, and low in non-fiber carbs. Eating organic and grass-fed is also important, as commonly used pesticides like glyphosate cause mitochondrial damage

**When you eat:** Daily intermittent fasting tends to be the easiest to adhere to, but any fasting schedule that you will consistently follow will work

**Exercise,** with high intensity interval exercises being the most effective

## COMMON QUESTIONS ABOUT AUTOPHAGY

### But when and why do cells die?

Some cells can get damaged due to external factors, like injury or poison or infections. So when you get a cut on your finger, cells whose blood supply gets cut-off, die. This is called Necrosis.

But some cells don't just die, they commit suicide.

Yes, cells kill themselves. Nothing external happens. Just that the cell becomes damaged due to excessive wear and tear, and the body decides its time is up. This process is called Apoptosis. And as macabre as it sounds, apoptosis is key to living a healthy life.

When a fetus is taking shape inside a mother's womb, it's feet are webbed. Slowly, the webbing disappears and we get distinct fingers. The cells in the webbing die voluntarily. Apoptosis. Our brains create millions of neurons at first. But only some of the neurons organise into neural pathways that become thoughts and memories. The rest die voluntarily. Apoptosis. Think of your body as a equipment-rental company.

Millions of cells that make it up, being the equipment it rents out. We, both biologically and philosophically, are just tenants in our bodies. And we have a contract with this company. So whenever we need to perform a task, the company lends us a certain number of specific machinery built for the task at hand. Want to lift a cup? The body mobilises muscular cells in your fingers and performs the task. Want to solve a hard problem? The body mobilises neural networks in the brain and supports you.

Want to run a marathon? The body hates you, but mobilises everything from muscle fibers to 'persistence' neural networks in the brain to help you scrape through. Now, due to prolonged use this equipment, like any equipment, goes through wear & tear. It becomes damaged and isn't able to reliably perform its assigned task.

But the body takes its contract very seriously. If you've been keeping your end of the bargain and giving it clean fuel for its equipment (aka food and exercise), it wants to ensure you get the right service everytime. And it can't guarantee that with damaged cells. So it does continuous quality checks on its entire fleet. The equipment (cells) that it finds are beyond repair, are decommissioned (killed). Apoptosis. The ones that can be fixed and made brand new, are sent in for repair. Sub-cellular repair. Autophagy.

**What turns off autophagy?**

Eating. Glucose, insulin (or decreased glucagon) and proteins all turn off this self-cleaning process. And it doesn't take much. Even a small amount of amino acid (leucine) could stop autophagy cold. So this process of autophagy is unique to fasting – something not found in simple caloric restriction or dieting.

**So when autophagy happens, is it just happening all over my body, everywhere?**

Basically, with a notable exception: Fasting appears to induce autophagy in most organs (like the liver, muscle, and pancreas), but "not in the brain."

**Are there any benefits of autophagy that sound too good to be true but you want to include them anyway, because you never know?**

Well, it sort of all sounds too good to be true, this incredibly easy way to just clean up internal problems but I especially like the vague idea that autophagy could be good for the complexion and potentially for skin diseases like psoriasis.

## Can autophagy be harmful?

Autophagy has been described as a "double-edged sword" for its seeming ability to both "exacerbate or mitigate injury."

Fasting in general can contribute to the development of gallstones, which can develop when bile stored in the gallbladder hardens into stonelike matter.

Fasting in general is also not recommended for underweight people, pregnant people, children, and the very elderly.

## Could fasting to induce autophagy be considered an eating disorder?

Not inherently, although excessive fasting to induce autophagy could overlap with anorexia. Many people fast for benefits beyond weight control, though, including disease prevention, muscle retention, and mental clarity.

## Can you fast to induce autophagy too much, or too frequently?

Yes. There are no exact rules or recommendations (yet?), but researchers agree that extended fasting for autophagy, like going for 36, 48, or even 72 hours without food is something that healthy people should do at most 2 or 3 times a year, and only after conferring with a doctor.

**Is there a way to know for sure whether or not autophagy is happening in my own body? Is there a way to measure it?**

Not yet. Measuring autophagy in humans, or measuring "autophagic flux" is tricky, because it involves the rising and falling ratios of certain tiny proteins (like the protein LC3 and its variants).

There's no such thing as an "autophagometer," for instance, and a 2017 study noted that it's "practically impossible to monitor autophagy properly in humans." In the meantime, you can measure things like glucose and ketones, which are affected by fasting. (And LC3 levels can be compared on a protein-identifying Western blot, or immunoblot, blood test.)

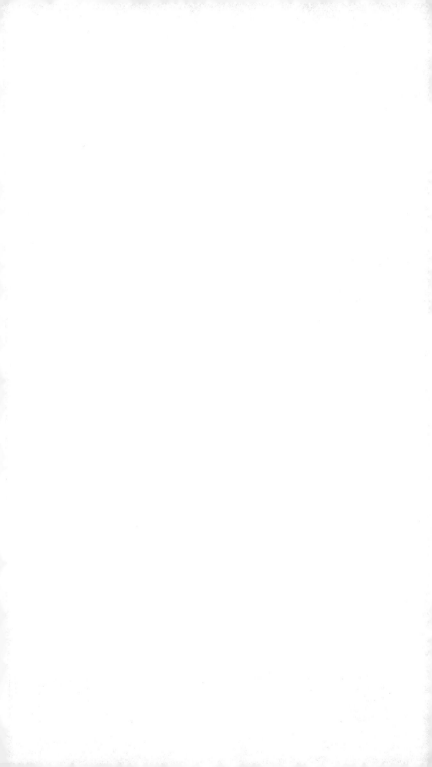

CPSIA information can be obtained
at www.ICGtesting.com
Printed in the USA
FFHW021248041019
55414684-61157FF